Lucy's Blue Ribbon

Lucy's Blue Ribbon

A SISTER'S PROMISE

Njeri G. Moore

Copyright © 2017 Njeri G. Moore
All rights reserved.

ISBN: 1541040082
ISBN-13: 9781541040083
Library of Congress Control Number: 2016920705
CreateSpace Independent Publishing Platform
North Charleston, South Carolina

Lucy's story told in this book is true. The conversations come from the author's recollection, though they are not written word-for-word. Some names have been changed to protect the privacy of individuals.

*For my hero, Esther Wawira Gathungu, my mami; without your love, sacrifice,
hard work, and compassion, I would not exist. You are forever in me.*

Contents

Acknowledgments

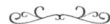

MY DEEPEST GRATITUDE GOES TO my friend Greg Pryor, my first reader and editor. This book could not have been completed without your encouragement; I am proud to call you and Ann my friends, and I love you. To my second reader and editor, Doris McBryde, who reviewed the completed manuscript and encouraged me to get it published, thank you so much.

I am grateful to my girlfriends: Sonya Thorne, who believed in me when I didn't believe in myself; Diane Fauntleroy, whose shoulder I have cried on more times than I can count; Nicole Moore, who reminded me to pick up where I left off whenever I stopped writing; and Tamara Long, Rae Mbugua, Rachel Cason, Pam Arungah, and Donna Marie, who have listened without judgment, comforted me, and encouraged me to tell Lucy's story as she would have wanted it told. I love you, my sister-friends.

When I was a child, my mother taught me that nothing matters more than loving and being loved by family. Thank you so much, Mami, Baba, Shiku, Gloria, Nancy, Lydiah, Jeff, Julie, Nina, Koki, Waititu, Ian, Ethan, Eli, Zeke, Nisey, Jude, Amaru, Nesta, Tata Ruguru, Tata Thiguku, and my extended family; your love surrounds me and keeps me pushing to do better, always; I love you. My daughters, Ethel and Jazmine: You are my pride, my joy, and my greatest achievement. Among other things, I am so proud of the curious and kind human beings you are. I love you so much. To my husband, Tony Moore, the love of my life and the kindest gentleman I know, who took time to understand and respect my Kenyan culture and loved my family from the beginning, words cannot express how grateful I am for you. I love you; I am the luckiest woman.

Last but certainly not least, I am grateful to all our family and friends who comforted us after Shiku's, Lucy's, and Mami's deaths; there are too many to mention here, but I know who you are. I am forever grateful to those who loved Lucy and did everything possible to make her wish come true. May God bless you always.

Introduction

LUCY WAS DIAGNOSED WITH STAGE IV colon cancer in September of 2009 at the age of thirty-four. This shocked her parents, siblings, extended family, and close friends, all of whom were still mourning the death of Shiku, Lucy's forty-two-year-old sister, who had passed away in January of 2008. After an extensive surgery in Okinawa, Japan, Lucy mustered the courage to reassure and comfort her family and, more importantly, refused to surrender to the disease. She did not wallow in self-pity; she believed she could fight the disease and beat the rather intimidating odds. During the fight, Lucy kept busy by using her creative genius to raise money for colon-cancer research and support children and family in Kenya. Lucy refused to be the helpless victim of an unfaithful, emotionally abusive marriage and instead focused on living her life consciously and purposefully every single day. Lucy, an avid writer, kept journals, which she confided to her sisters contained material to tell her personal story. It was her ambition to write a book using those journals, and that ambition became both her motivation and inspiration. She would tease her sisters with bits and pieces about the content but told them they needed to wait until she was done.

Lucy fought a brave battle throughout the years, but in August of 2014, Lucy learned from her oncologist that the cancer was terminal and that she did not have long to live. She called in her sisters, Njeri, Gloria, and Lydiah, and made her wishes known to them. Among other things, she wanted to be buried in her ancestral land next to her sister Shiku in Kenya. She wanted her charity work of helping children in Kenya by providing school supplies and other support to continue. She asked that her sisters continue to educate people about colon cancer by telling her story and asking that her journals be used. Unfortunately, when Lucy passed away, her sisters were denied the manuscript and the journals, even though she had bequeathed them in her last will and testament. Nil, her estranged husband, refused to honor her wishes.

After her death, Lucy's sisters fought and won the right to bury her where she wanted, next to her sister in Kenya. The family later embarked on a project to honor Lucy's wishes. They formed "Lucy's Blue Ribbon," a project that strives to give hope to those who feel hopeless through encouragement and financial and emotional support while drawing on the teachings that Lucy left behind regarding hope, faith, strength, courage, love, and compassion. At the time of this writing, the family has provided backpacks and other school supplies to more than fifty children and has pledged to continue helping school children achieve academic excellence through mentoring and providing basic school needs so children can stay in school.

This book tells Lucy's story based on conversations, observations, and experiences as witnessed mainly by her sister Njeri with input from her sisters Gloria and Lydiah. Lucy was known to speak her mind, because she believed holding grudges was wrong. Njeri realized she did not need Lucy's journals or the transcripts to tell her story, as she knew it well. This book fulfills one of Lucy's wishes. Some proceeds from this book will go toward colon-cancer research and Lucy's Blue Ribbon, starting with those children Lucy cared about in Kenya.

Lucy endured colon cancer with great fortitude. She knew who she was and what she wanted, and she would not let anyone or anything change her. She had love and empathy for her fellow human beings; she found humor and happiness in little things; she always challenged herself with new business ideas, and she was always forgiving. Lucy's story inspires those who loved her to stand up even when life knocks them down. Hopefully, it does the same for others who hear it for the first time.

CHAPTER 1

Please Let Me Go

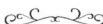

LUCY HAD BEEN AT THE Fort Belvoir hospital in the same sixth-floor room for three weeks due to bowel obstruction, a complication from advanced colon cancer. She was supposed to leave the hospital on the morning of September 5, but her situation became more complicated the day before. Lucy had insisted that her sister Njeri spend Thursday and Friday nights with her. Throughout her stay, Lucy had been chatty, telling jokes like she always did and being opinionated as usual. On these two nights, she mostly slept but occasionally would wake up, asking how long she had been sleeping and if Njeri were OK. She seemed more concerned about her sister than herself.

"You need to get some food," Lucy told Njeri.

"I am not hungry, sis," Njeri responded. "Besides, it's late anyway, and I already had dinner."

Shortly after midnight on Friday, September 5, 2014, the nurse walked into the room to take Lucy's vitals and noticed that her oxygen level was low and her blood pressure very high. A few minutes later, there was a team of doctors in the room, examining her. Njeri left the room, nervously shaking, not wanting Lucy to see that she was deathly scared. After composing herself, she walked in to find Lucy laughing, telling the doctors that it tickled when they touched her stomach. At 1:00 a.m., a decision to take her into ICU so they could monitor her more closely was made.

As Lucy was wheeled away, she called out to her sister, "Njeri, grab my iPhone and keep it with you no matter what." Njeri saw the pink-cased iPhone next to the bed, picked it up, and put it in her pocket.

The room was ready when they arrived in ICU. While the nurse was settling Lucy in, Njeri went to the waiting room to call Nil, Lucy's husband, to give him an update. As she walked back into the room, for the first time, Njeri saw fear in Lucy's eyes.

They hugged tightly, and Lucy whispered to her sister, "Don't leave me." Njeri assured her that she would stay in the room with her, and Lucy smiled and shortly fell asleep.

A few minutes before 4:00 a.m., Lucy opened her eyes, looking to see who was in the room. Njeri was sitting on a chair beside the bed, singing the last song they had sang, a popular Kenyan song their mother had taught them when she visited the United States:

"Upendo wa Mungu kweli, ni wa ajabu (God's love truly is amazing)
Upendo wa Mungu kweli, ni wa ajabu (God's love truly is amazing*)*
Waweza kwenda mbele (It goes forward)
Waweza kwenda nyuma (It goes backward)
Waweza kwenda juu (It goes up)
Waweza kwenda chini (It goes down)
Upande upande kwa mataifa yote (It goes side to side, all around the nations)
Upande upande kwa mataifa yote. (It goes side by side, all around the nations)

Lucy smiled, reached for her sister's hand, and quietly said in Kikuyu, *"Njeri, reke thii,"* meaning "Njeri, please let me go." Her sister was not sure she heard clearly, so she asked her to repeat. This time, Lucy was loud and clear.

"Please, let me go!"

"Are you sure you are ready, sis?" Njeri did not know what else to say.

"Yes. Call Mami, Baba, and all in Kenya so I can say good-bye. Also, tell Gloria, Lydiah, and the kids to come over now so I can see them."

Njeri immediately called Gloria and Lydiah, asking them to hurry up; she then called her two daughters and asked them to get ready to be picked up by their aunt Gloria and come to the hospital.

Lucy seemed to have a burst of energy. She asked the nurse to raise the bed a little higher and waited as Njeri called their parents in Kenya. Their mother, who they all called Mami, was the first on the line. Njeri explained that Lucy's condition had worsened and that the doctors said they could do nothing else, then handed the phone to Lucy. Njeri heard Mami crying, asking Lucy not to leave her.

Lucy kept repeating in Kikuyu, "Please let me go, Mami."

After a while Mami's crying stopped. Lucy calmly assured Mami that she would see her in heaven. She also told her that after her soul left, Njeri would bring her body home for burial so Mami could say good-bye. Mami handed the phone to their father, who they called Baba.

Lucy said in Kikuyu, "Baba, I am ready to go." Baba said a prayer and told Lucy that God's will would be done. Next, Lucy spoke to their only brother, Jeff, telling him she loved him and asking that he pass her love to her sister Nancy and all the nephews and nieces. Lucy's final words to Mami and Baba and Jeff were "I love you."

Lucy slowly drifted back to sleep after the conversations with her family in Kenya. Shortly after, Nil, her husband, came into the room with a suitcase and demanded that Njeri leave the room so he could speak to his wife. He started to draw the curtains as Njeri was leaving, but the nurse didn't allow it. Minutes later, he hurriedly left the ICU and went into the sixth-floor room where Lucy had been staying for three weeks. Nil took her laptop, which had the transcript of the book she was writing, her journals, inspirational books, magazines, everything except the flowers and plants that family and friends had left Lucy. He was upset to learn that Lucy had given Njeri the authority to handle the end-of-life decision, so he was not allowed to "pull the plug." He left the hospital never to talk to Lucy again and did not return until three hours after her death.

Lucy's sister Lydiah, her husband, Mike, and the boys, Ethan, Eli, and Ezekiel arrived from Maryland shortly after 6:00 a.m. Her sister Gloria, nephew Ian, and Njeri's daughters, Ethel and Jazmine, followed a few minutes later. They visited Lucy in intervals, and she told each one of them that she loved them. At some point, it became difficult for her to breathe, so when her nieces Ethel and Jazmine came in to see her, she gestured that she was stinking and gave a big smile, which they all laughed at. An hour or so later, Lucy could no longer breathe on her own, and the doctors said they had to intubate her. When they brought her back, the doctors said she was no longer in pain and that the family could stay in the room with her while she transitioned. Njeri asked the doctors to call the chaplain who had been visiting Lucy for the past three weeks. Njeri called her husband, Tony, to let him know that it was time. She also called James, a longtime family friend, to let him know. Both James and the chaplain arrived within an hour of being notified. For a few hours, the sisters held her hands, prayed, and sang.

The only way Njeri knew that it was midmorning of September, 6, 2014, was by looking at her watch. Everything surrounding her was surreal. Laying on the high, raised bed at the Fort Belvoir Hospital Intensive Care Unit, Lucy was hooked to several different machines. The ICU doctors induced sedation to reduce the pain, and Lucy could no longer speak. Njeri sat beside the bed, slowly massaging Lucy's hand as if to soothe her. Her other sisters Gloria and Lydiah sat close, each touching a part of Lucy's body. Mike, Lydiah's husband, and James were also in the room, joined by the hospital Chaplain Nobles, who had brought with him a few Christian hymnals. The room was filled with quiet singing, the beeping of the heart monitor, the repetitive sound made by the blood pressure monitor, the nasogastric (NG) tube suctioning every so often, the breathing machines, and all the other machines that Lucy was hooked to. Somehow, even with everything going on, there was a sense of peace and calmness in the brightly lit room. Lucy seemed as though she was listening intently as her chest rose slowly up and down. Every few minutes, the nurses and the doctors would stop by to check on her. Everyone in the room knew it was just a matter of time. The doctors had assured them that Lucy would peacefully pass away knowing her loved ones surrounded her. She had fought for more than five years and outlasted all earlier prognoses. When she was diagnosed with stage IV colon cancer, she had been given two years to live, yet she lived five meaningful years.

CHAPTER 2

Lucy Growing up in Kenya

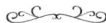

ON THE NIGHT OF TUESDAY, July 29, 1975, Baba burst into to the small house in Athi-River town, where he lived with Mami and their four girls. He excitedly announced that there was a new member of the family. The girls woke up confused and sleepy, as they had gone to bed a few hours earlier in order to be ready for school the following day. Njeri, a curious, happy-go-lucky girl, was the oldest at eleven years old; Baba had named her after his mother. Nine-year-old Shiku was more mature and thoughtful than her older sister but preferred to say she was ten because she was turning double digits in a couple of months. They had named Shiku after Mami's mother. Gloria, known by the sisters as Waruguru, a skinny, talkative, long-haired daughter, had just turned eight; she was named after Baba's oldest sister, who had raised him after he was orphaned. Nancy was quiet but demanded attention, and as she had been the youngest of the siblings for six years, Baba spoiled her.

"I love my girls," Baba yelled as he made sure all the girls were awake to get details of his good news. Baba had brought with him *nyama choma* (barbeque meat), a rare treat that usually happened on a pay day Friday. It was obvious that he was a little tipsy as he kept repeating over again how beautiful the new baby girl was and how much he loved his girls. "We named her Lucy after your aunt Lucia," Baba announced. There was no mistaking that he was a happy man.

Baba looked and sounded different than other men in town. He wore dress pants and a sports jacket to both work and bars and spoke intellectually.

He was a smart, charming man who knew how to tell a story; he drew attention when he spoke. It was not surprising that he met Mami a few years after he graduated from high school and swept her off her feet. Mami became pregnant, was kicked out of school, and never allowed to return even after she had Njeri. In the small town where they lived, other men laughed at Baba because he did not have a son. The idea that no one would carry on his name or that no one would inherit the land that he had inherited from his father because he didn't have a son was ridiculous to Baba. He often said that his girls had as many rights as boys to live and die in his inherited land,

"A child is a child," he always said.

Around social places in the small town of Athi-River, men would joke that Baba was crazy to think that one of his girls would get the ancestral land or carry on the family name after he was gone. No one would dare say this to his face; a story was told of how Baba, who stood at five feet five inches tall, had beaten a man almost twice his size in a bar when the man told him that all women at some point became prostitutes willingly or unwillingly. The man told Baba that he should be prepared to have five prostitutes in his house at some point. Baba lost his temper and broke the man's nose. However, for his own reasons, Baba always reminded his girls that the biggest inheritance they would get from him was an education, something most men in Kenya at the time did not believe. Mami, on the other hand, did not speak much but led by example.

At five feet eight inches, Mami was taller than Baba by three inches. She was a no-nonsense woman who did not mince words. "You become someone's slave when he or she realizes you need them for everything. You become a slave when you let someone or anything control you," Mami would say. She meant what she said, even when it seemed trivial; when she started working outside the house, she had extra money to buy soda every day. For a month, she came home with several bottles of Fanta and Coca-Cola for the girls. One evening when the girls asked her if she forgot the soda, she said, "We were becoming slaves of the soda, so from now on, no more soda every day. You can get it once in a while."

Mami was a fiercely independent woman who was obviously in charge. Men and women in the town revered her and came to her for advice. All the neighborhood children respected her and affectionately called her Mami. It was known that if you were hungry, Mami would feed you without hesitating, and so, as a result, her small house was always full. Mami was at work when she went into labor with Lucy. She took a taxi without letting her coworkers know and asked the nurses to contact Baba only when they told her she couldn't go back home, since she was already dilated. A few hours after Mami was admitted, little Lucy was born. Four days later, Mami came home with a chubby, curly-haired, dark-skinned baby who everyone fell in love with.

Each of the sisters played a specific role with baby Lucy after Mami hired a house girl to take care of Lucy and returned to work. Njeri, the oldest, was like a mother hen protecting her chick. She allowed no one to go near the baby unless they knew how to hold her. Shiku played the role of caretaker and helped change diapers and bathe her. Gloria made sure that Lucy ate all her food. Nancy, the six-year-old, was a playmate who always kept Lucy entertained. The girls' childhood was full of fun and joy. They all got along fine and were one another's best friends. They spent hours playing and being creative. Baba's and Mami's small house was where parents sent their children when they needed tutoring or something to eat. The girls had no clue that they were poor. They learned very early to have fun together. Mami impressed upon them that having love for one another and looking out for one another was central to happiness.

At age six, Lucy started attending Moi Avenue Primary School in Nairobi, which was twenty-eight kilometers from Athi-River. Shortly after, one by one the older sisters left home for boarding school. In July of 1984, when Lucy was a few days shy of her ninth birthday, Mami gave birth to another girl, who they named Lydiah after Mami's sister who had taken her in when she became pregnant as a young girl. Three years later in 1987, Mami and Baba finally had their son, Ayub, named after Baba's father; the girls were asked to pick his middle name, and they agreed on Jeff. By that time, all the older sisters had left home so, naturally, Lucy became the big sister, a role she took very seriously until her dying day.

For Lucy, the happy-go-lucky life changed one afternoon during the August holidays when she was thirteen years old. She fed her siblings Lydiah and Jeff and laid them down for an afternoon nap. She looked outside the flat where they now lived and saw her friends congregated, chatting excitedly. She knew that she had an hour to socialize before the children work up. She shut the door behind her and headed down the stairs to join her friends. As she reached the corridor, a man who had recently moved into the neighborhood grabbed her, dragged her into the house, and raped her. He threatened to do it again if she told on him and told her she should not have left her siblings in the house alone.

The traumatic ordeal left Lucy confused and terrified. Lucy went back in the house, crying, and took a long shower. She got rid of the bloody underwear and laid in bed, not knowing what to do. When Mami came home, she noticed that something was wrong, but Lucy did not tell her what it was. For a long time, Lucy was afraid to leave the house by herself. She no longer went out to play with her friends and would not let Jeff and Lydiah out of her sight unless Mami, Baba, or one of her older sisters accompanied them. On the days she was out of school, instead of going outside to socialize with other children her age, Lucy would spend hours cleaning the house and finding projects to occupy her time. She questioned her self-worth and felt that she was at fault for the man raping her. It wasn't until years later that Lucy told her sisters, but it was too late. She was never the same person; the rape had changed her. During this time, Lucy developed a closer relationship with Mami. She noticed that Mami was always helping other people. Women who did not have money to buy food for their children stopped by the house to borrow from Mami who gave joyfully. Mami would talk about something she wanted, but when she got the money, she would instead buy shoes for a neighbor's child or give the money to a family in need. Lucy wanted to know why Mami was so generous so she asked her. Mami's response was, "I have everything I need. They need shoes, food and other things more than I do. I've been on the receiving end. I know that being able to give is a blessing from God and it makes me happy".

While being reclusive, Lucy took an interest in people Mami was helping. She would skip lunch to give the money to those she felt needed it. She tapped into her inner self and discovered that she loved how she felt watching others smile when she did them a favor. Around the time of Lucy's rape, Baba was laid off from a job he had worked for almost two decades and moved to the countryside to farm, leaving Mami as the sole bread winner. Lucy helped

Mami with expenses, getting up early in the morning to make chapati (flat bread) to sell, a job she took seriously. After a few months, Mami felt that Lucy needed to devote more time to school in order to pass her primary school and be accepted into a good high school. Mami asked Njeri, who had recently become a flight attendant with Pan American World Airways and moved into her own apartment in Nairobi, if Lucy could stay with her. During her last year in primary school, Lucy moved in with Njeri, passed her exams, and was admitted to Ngara Girls High School in Nairobi.

While attending high school, Lucy took turns staying with her older sisters who, were employed and lived independently. Once again, they each played their childhood roles. In 1990, Njeri immigrated to the United States. She made a promise to Lucy that once settled, she would send for her. Lucy did well in high school, but like many students, she was not admitted to one of the two public universities everyone competed to get into. The few private universities were very expensive. The wealthy Kenyans sent their children abroad to attend universities. This was not an option for Lucy, as her family could not afford it. However, Lucy stayed hopeful because she had faith that her sister Njeri would keep her promise, as she always did.

Lucy spent the year and a half after graduation reacquainting herself with childhood friends. She slowly started socializing and hanging out with them and soon started dating. She still helped care for her sister Lydiah and her brother, Jeff, and liked a couple of boys. She started feeling like her old self before the rape but refused to go anywhere alone. In one case, Lucy's relationship became serious when one of the boys who, at twenty, was two years older than her came to visit a relative in Nairobi and asked her to marry him. Lucy decided to elope because she knew no one would approve of it. As soon as Lucy left Nairobi for Mombasa, Mami called Gloria's fiancé, John, who was a police officer, and asked him to find Lucy and the boy. John drove almost five hundred kilometers from Nairobi to Mombasa and found the boy's family, who took him to where Lucy was now getting ready to settle into her new life as a would-be wife. Whatever John did left the boy scared; Lucy was ordered into the car, and they drove back to Nairobi, stopping once to get something to eat. Two months later, shortly before her twentieth birthday, Lucy was on her way to Oceanside, California to join her sister Njeri.

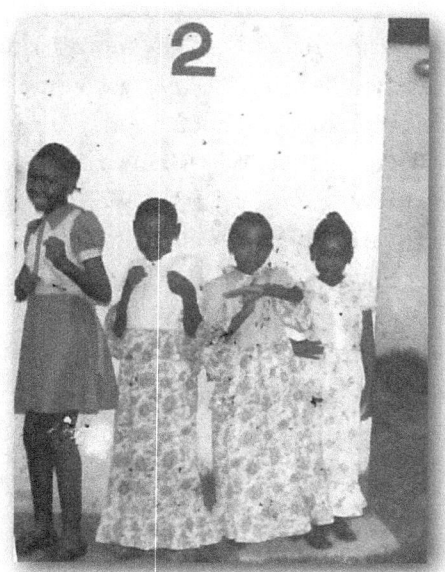

Njeri, Shiku, Gloria and Nancy shortly before Lucy was born

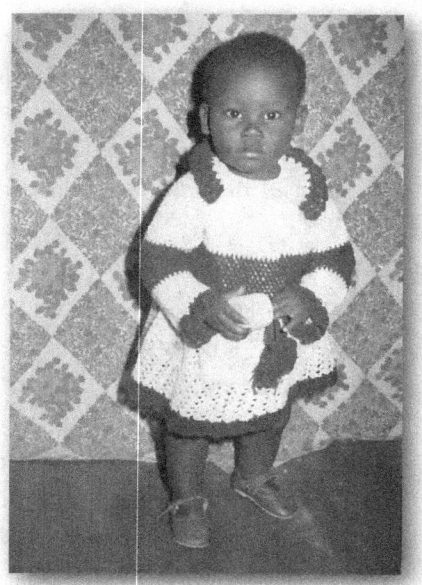

Baby Lucy at 18 months

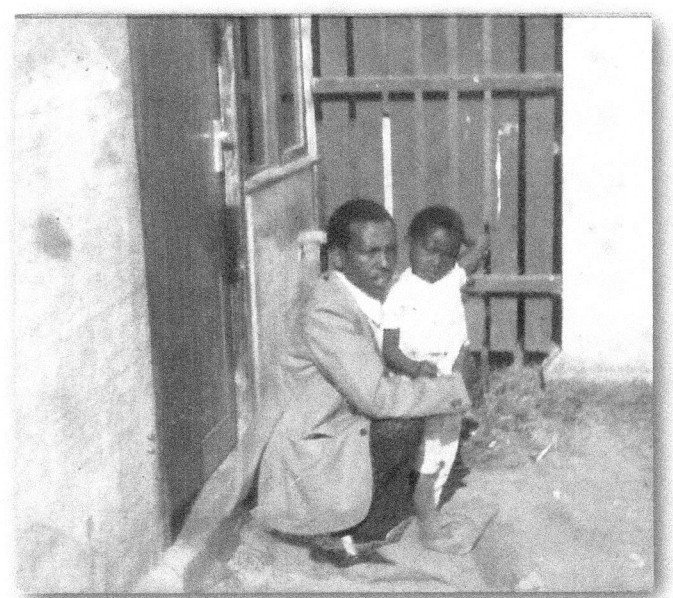

Lucy, 2 years old and Baba

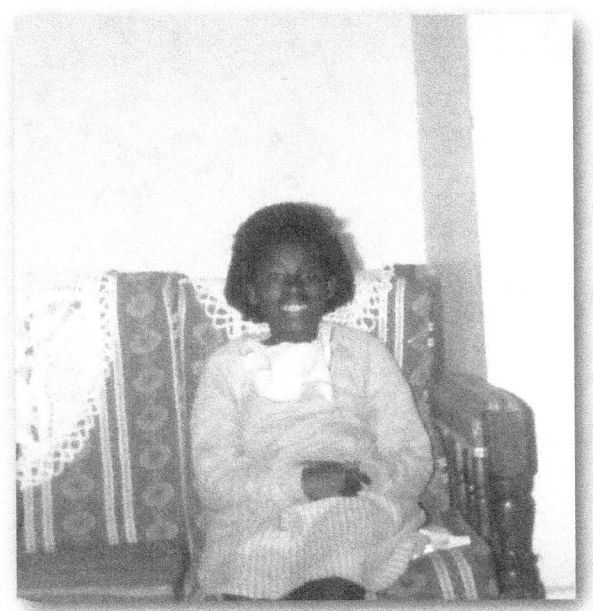

Lucy at age 10

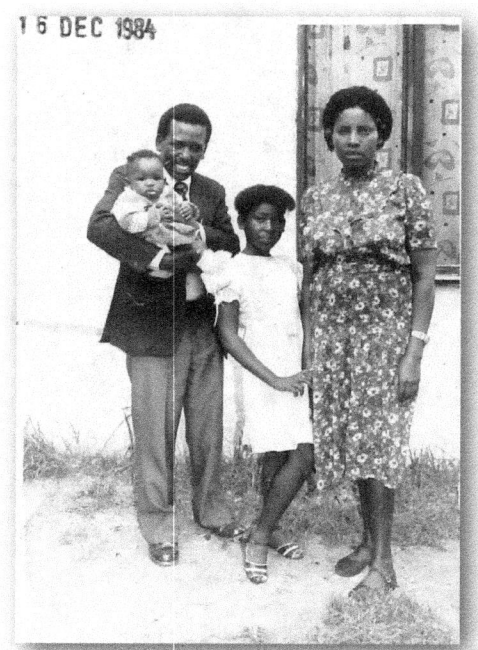

Baba holding Lydiah, Lucy and Mami

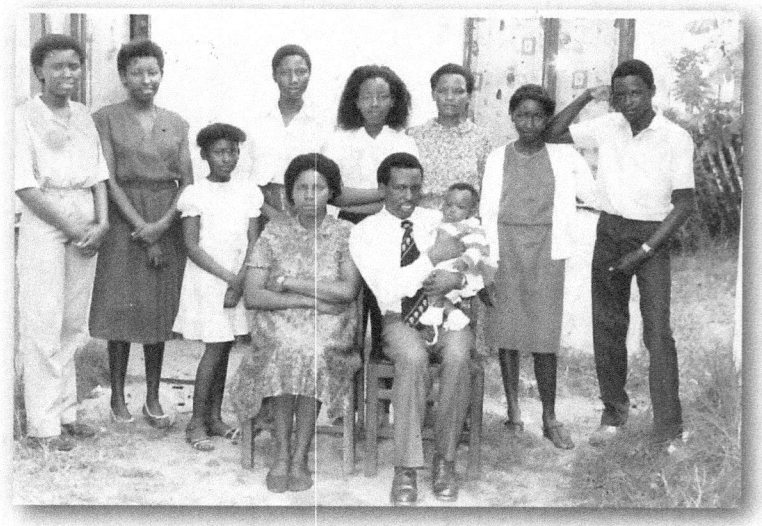

The family and cousins before Jeff was born

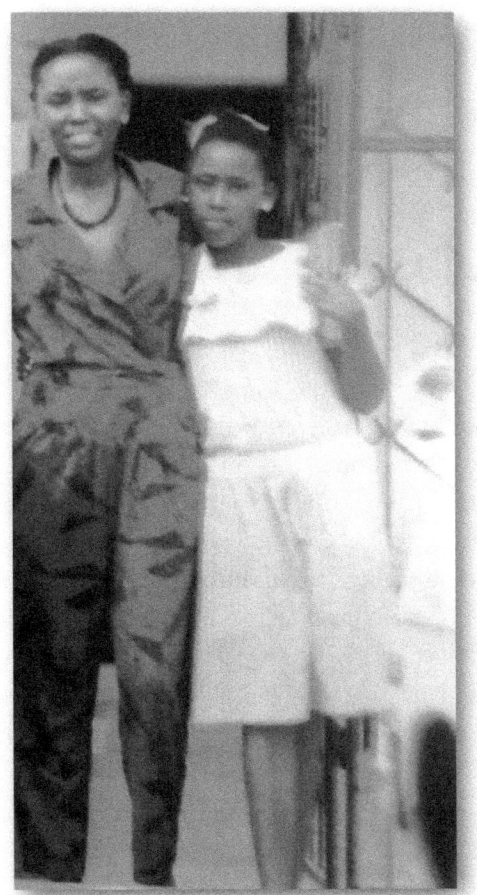

Lucy at age 12 with Njeri

CHAPTER 3

Welcome to America

LUCY TRAVELED FROM NAIROBI THROUGH London to reach the Los Angeles airport. After clearing customs and immigration, Lucy took a small shuttle aircraft to San Diego airport. It was a perfect seventy-three degrees Fahrenheit one early spring afternoon when Njeri walked toward the small plane parked on the tarmac. Several passengers disembarked, each picking their small pieces of luggage, which were lined up next to the plane. Njeri wondered if her sister had missed the flight; as she started walking toward the gate agent, she caught a glimpse of Lucy who had a big smile on her face. The two sisters ran toward each other and hugged, laughing and crying at the same time; there was no mistaking how happy they were to see each other. For Njeri, it was a promise kept and the joy of knowing she would have a sibling in America. For Lucy, it was a dream come true.

Njeri had not seen her sister in two years and was surprised to see how much weight she had lost. At five feet four inches, Lucy was a size 0–2. She wore a white shirt and a pair of green jeans. Her hair was cut into the mullet style, which was referred to as the "business in front and party in back" hairstyle. She carried a small black backpack. The two sisters proceeded to baggage claim. After a short wait, Lucy pulled a small suitcase from the carousel and said that she had only one extra set of clothing; everything else was the coffee, tea, and other gifts Mami had given her to bring her sister.

The drive to Camp Pendleton Marine Corp Base where Njeri's husband was stationed as a marine took less than an hour. Lucy was exhausted from the long trip, so she took a long shower, ate, and went to sleep. The following morning, the sisters had breakfast and spent the rest of the day reminiscing about their childhood, family, and everything else. Lucy bonded immediately with her four-year-old niece, Ethel, who excitedly held her aunt's hand and would not let go.

After dinner, Ethel, who was sitting across from Lucy at the dinner table, stared curiously, then asked, "Aunt Lucy, why are some of your teeth brown? Did you forget to brush them?"

Lucy burst out laughing while Njeri and her husband, Tony, stared at Ethel, disapproving of the question.

"No, Ethel," Lucy responded. "When your mother and your aunts were young, Baba found a job in a town called Athi-River for work. The town had a water treatment facility where they added too much fluoride. All the children born in that town or who still had their baby teeth now have discolored teeth. It is called fluorosis."

"I like white teeth. Can you make yours white?"

"I hope so," Lucy replied.

Njeri and Tony decided that getting the teeth taken care of was a priority in order for Lucy to feel comfortable. After researching, Njeri found out that senior students at UCLA School of Dentistry had a program where they would take cases as part of their learning for a small fee. Njeri made the phone call, and Lucy was given an appointment for consultation. For two months, Njeri and Lucy made regular early-morning trips on Interstate 5 from Camp Pendleton to UCLA. The procedures were painful, and at some point, Lucy wanted it to stop. Although the student dentist did not fix the problem entirely, the treatment made Lucy less conscious of her teeth.

Lucy was eager to earn her own money by working, so she told a neighbor that she knew how to braid hair using extensions. The neighbor promised to pay Lucy fifty dollars if she braided her daughter's hair. One day when Njeri arrived from work, she found Lucy struggling to braid the hair; she had no idea how to do it. Njeri ended up braiding the little girl's hair and did not do a good job, either. The neighbor never paid the fifty dollars. This was the end of Lucy's hair braiding idea. Her next job would be from yet another neighbor.

Njeri and Tony had developed a close relationship with their next door neighbors James and Shandra. Like Tony, James was also in the marine corp. The couples spent weekend hours together eating, drinking, and having a great time. Occasionally, the couples hired a babysitter to watch their children Ashanti and Tre both close in age with Ethel. Recently, James had decided to start a business delivering newspapers for extra cash. He thought he would move faster if he had Lucy running the paper to the front door or mailbox while he focused on driving. For a few months, Lucy and James delivered newspapers, and James paid her on time. Lucy wired her first paycheck of sixty dollars to Mami, who called Lucy back a few days later, expressing her gratitude and blessings. Ironically, the phone call cost more than the sixty dollars. After a few months, and due to work commitment, James stopped delivering papers, so Lucy had to find another job.

Fortunately, Shandra, James's wife, worked for the *Marine Corps Community Services* (MCCS) in the Administrative Office at Camp Pendleton. Her office was responsible for recruiting and staffing for different programs aimed at improving the lives of the marines and their families. Shandra told Lucy to apply for a position at one of the stores as a sales clerk or a cashier. Prior to the interview, Shandra took time to train Lucy on counting American money and giving the correct change. Lucy was hired at one of the stores, a job she held for ten years, performing multiple duties and responsibilities.

During her first year of working at the store, Lucy made lifelong friends and even went on a couple of dates with a young marine named Ed. Njeri liked Ed, but Lucy thought he was immature and inconsiderate. One evening, they went to dinner at Red Lobster in Oceanside. Lucy was not feeling well, so she had no appetite.

Ed asked her, "Aren't you going to eat this food? You know I am paying for it." Before Lucy answered, he started digging in her plate and finished all of his and her food. Lucy had only one piece of the cheesy bread.

Ed dropped Lucy at Njeri's house at 10:00 p.m. where she went straight to the kitchen to look for something to eat. When Njeri heard her, she asked, "Didn't you go out to dinner?"

"Njeri, if I tell you that Ed eats like a pig, you won't believe it. You have to see it for yourself; I am breaking up with him. He only thinks about himself," Lucy said.

"Invite him to dinner on Friday before you break up," Njeri suggested.

Lucy laughed and agreed.

Ed arrived at Njeri's house at 7:30 p.m. Njeri was serving fried chicken, Kenyan greens called *sukuma wiki*, and rice and beans. James was also invited; Shandra and the children were out of town visiting family. As a courtesy, Tony and Njeri asked the guests to serve themselves first. Ed took most of the chicken, and others had to share the remaining few pieces. Tony only had two pieces of chicken wings; Njeri had one. Lucy and Njeri were giggling every time they looked at Ed. He never lifted his head from the plate. The following day, Lucy told Ed that she could no longer see him.

Lucy loved her job at the military store. For the first time, she was consistently earning a paycheck. One evening, Njeri was supposed to pick Lucy up from work, but she was running late. Lucy told Njeri that her friend and a work colleague, Regina, would give her a ride. Regina was a beautiful, tall, shy girl the same age as Lucy, and she lived with her uncle, JV. Lucy told Njeri that she and Regina had something in common; they had survived a traumatic event from their childhoods. Lucy did not share with Njeri what that was for Regina.

JV and Regina dropped Lucy off, and Njeri asked them to join her for tea. JV hugged Njeri, and then followed her to the kitchen when she was preparing to make the tea. "Lucy, your big sister is as beautiful as you. Actually, I prefer a glass of water instead of tea if that's ok with you," JV said. The first impression Njeri got after meeting JV was that he was uninhibited. JV was stocky and stood almost six feet tall and looked racially ambiguous. He must have been in his late forties. He had long, slick hair and was wearing a gold chain. His shirt was unbuttoned, exposing the gold medallion, reminding Njeri of the rapper LL Cool J. He had a big smile, and his two bottom teeth were missing. Njeri would later learn that he was involved in an accident while repairing his car. During this meeting, Njeri found out that JV was a Creole from Louisiana. He loved to cook and occasionally invited friends over for dinner at his house. Njeri also learned that JV had previously been married, but his wife left him after a few years. Until recently, he had lived with his beloved cocker spaniel puppy, Camille. His niece, Regina, had asked if she could move to California to get a fresh start. JV had agreed to let her move in with him, since he had a big three-bedroom house. The fact that JV had taken his niece in impressed Njeri. After Regina and JV left, Njeri confided to Lucy that she thought JV was a little unguarded in his conversation, considering this was their first time meeting.

JV and Regina become Lucy's ride to and from work. On weekends, Lucy would visit with Regina and sometimes spend the night. Njeri was happy to see that Lucy had met a good friend until one day when, after JV dropped her off, Lucy announced to Njeri that he had asked to marry her.

Njeri reacted by laughing and joking, "He is old enough to be your father."

Lucy did not find this funny. "He is; I think I love him," she said. "I told him he has to ask you first before I can say yes."

"You must be out of your mind. There is no way you will marry that man. I am ordering you to stop seeing him effective immediately." Njeri stormed out of the room, disappointed that Lucy would even consider marrying JV. The days that followed were uncomfortable for both sisters. Njeri refused to discuss JV's proposal and even became belligerent toward Lucy. JV and Regina were no longer welcome, and Lucy was forbidden to see him. Lucy, who thought of her sister more like a mother, refused to engage in any arguments. She could longer take Njeri's nagging, so she packed up one day while Njeri was at work and moved in with Regina and JV. This was just a couple of months before Njeri's big birthday party. That evening, Njeri called Mami, requesting she talk some sense into Lucy. Mami's response was that Njeri needed to let Lucy grow up just as Mami had done with Njeri. She said that Lucy would learn from her own mistakes, if indeed they were. Njeri's pride would not allow her to apologize to her sister. Lucy refused to return and instead told Njeri that she had agreed to marry JV. She set the wedding date on Valentine's Day of the coming year.

Lucy came to Njeri's birthday party. She had JV drop her off a few blocks away from the house. She was very quiet and mostly interacted with Tony and Ethel and barely said anything to her sister. When Njeri asked her to come back to the house, Lucy said that would never happen and left the party shortly after. It took a while, but Njeri finally came to her senses after Tony, Mami, and Shandra called on her stubbornness and unwillingness to accept that Lucy was now a grown woman who did not need her protection. Mami and Baba gave JV their blessing, and Njeri was pleased that Lucy forgave her and asked her to be her maid of honor.

The wedding was held at JV's house. The guest list of twenty to thirty people included James, Shandra, and their children Ashanti and Tre. Ethel was the flower girl. Lucy wore a midlength white straight dress that hugged her butt and waistline. Her hair and makeup were on point; her six-inch white stiletto shoes made her legs longer. Baba had asked Tony to represent him in all things a father should do for his daughter since Baba could not make it to the wedding from Kenya. Tony took the role seriously and walked Lucy down the aisle, holding her hand tightly.

As Lucy walked into the room beaming, JV had two tear drops rolling down his cheeks. Njeri was feeling like an idiot as she realized her little sister was a grown woman in love.

By all accounts, Lucy's marriage to JV was happy for many years. They had challenges, which included Lucy being diagnosed with hypothyroidism and having to go through radiation treatment. Lucy had made it clear to JV that she would continue to support her family financially, and he was supportive of her position. When needed, they both worked two jobs to make things happen. Baba and Mami visited Oceanside and were happy that Lucy had found someone who loved and respected her. JV and Baba shared a common interest as craftsmen, fixing and building things.

Tony was transferred from Camp Pendleton to Brooklyn, New York, so in December of 1997, Njeri left her sister in California. Lucy and JV sponsored Lydiah, her youngest sister, when she graduated high school in Kenya to come to the United States and study at UCLA San Bernardino.

While working at the military store in Camp Pendleton, Lucy started classes at Mira Costa College to become a pharmacy technician. Her goal was to eventually become a pharmacist. She graduated as class valedictorian with a 4.0 GPA. During their marriage, Lucy and JV tried to have children but did not succeed. She made several doctors' visits, but they could not find any problems with her except that she had small fibroid tumors in her uterus. The doctors did not believe this would prevent conception. Lucy decided that she would not stress over getting pregnant and indeed if it happened, she would welcome it. Either way, she believed there were many children out in the world that needed parents.

For a long time, Lucy contemplated adopting a child from Kenya, but after researching, she realized that the process was not only costly but complicated. The Kenyan government took time vetting those interested in adopting Kenyan children. Apparently, there were people who pretended to adopt orphans from Kenya but their main intention was to traffic them as sex slaves or whatever they could benefit from. Lucy did not have the resources to go through the vigorous process. Instead, she continued helping children anonymously by sending money to Mami who would give to those children most in need. For Lucy and Mami, this was the most gratifying deed that kept them motivated; it was truly a common bond and their little secret.

After a year of college, Lucy's younger sister Lydiah transferred to a community college in order to save money. Shortly after, Lydiah met Mike and fell madly in love. JV and Lucy gave them a beautiful wedding where Lucy was the maid of honor. Lydiah and Mike moved to New York after their wedding so, once again, Lucy was in California without the family she was used to. After ten years of marriage, Lucy and JV had grown apart and decided to separate amicably. JV decided to move back to Louisiana. Lucy met Nil, whom she considered a nice guy, and decided to stay in California.

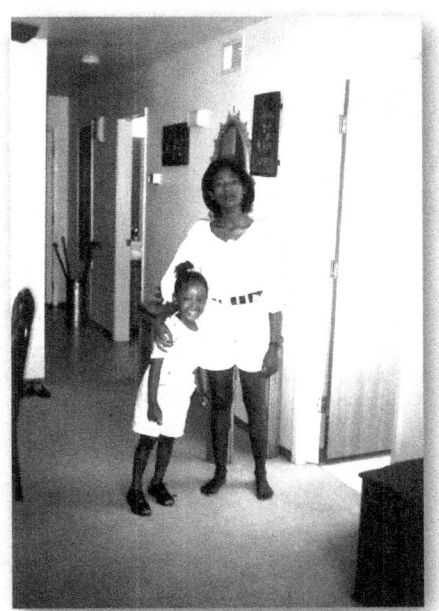

Lucy and Ethel; the picture was taken shortly after Lucy arrived in California.

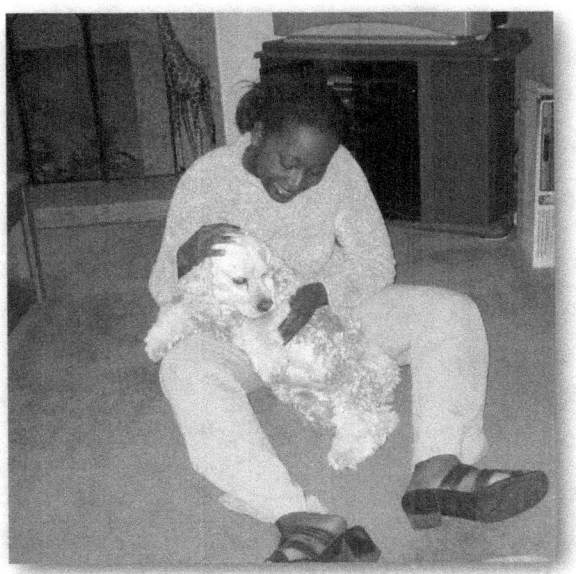

Lucy and JV's dog Camille

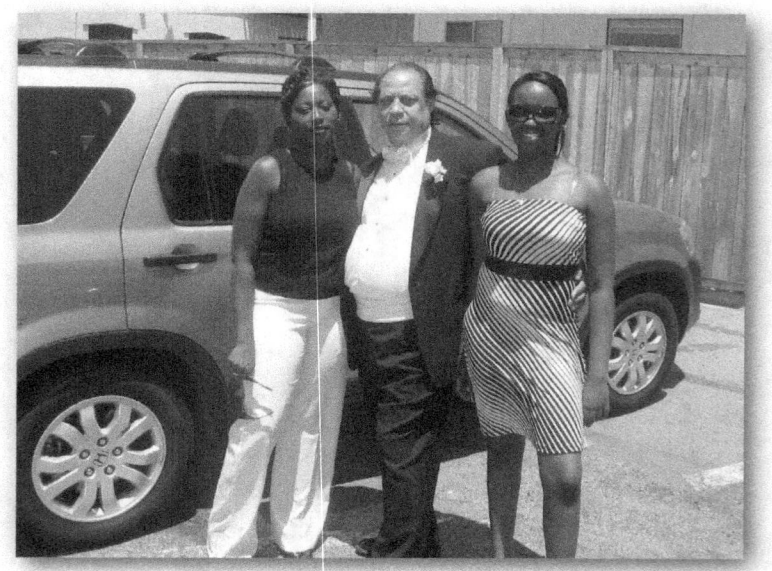

Lucy, JV and Lydiah

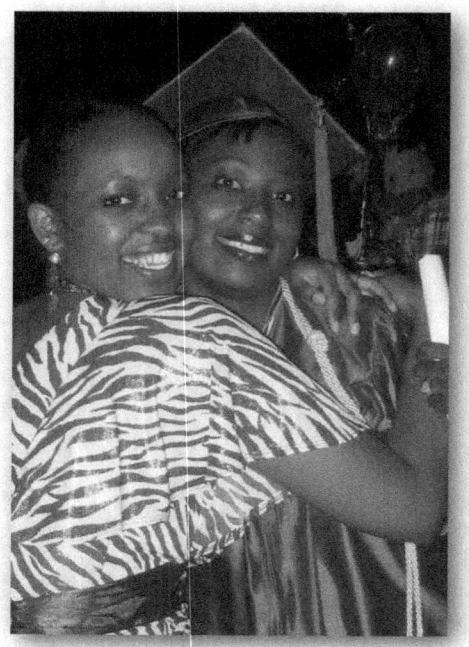

Lucy and Lydiah on graduation day

CHAPTER 4

Second Time Around

FOR MORE THAN A YEAR, Lucy had been planning on getting her own place. She and JV continued to live together and behaved more like roommates than a couple ready to divorce. They agreed not to rush through the divorce until they figured how to divide their assets and Lucy was financially ready to be on her own. She was now working two jobs: full-time as a pharmacy technician and part-time at the military store in Camp Pendleton. This was a stressful period, and Lucy found relief in the gym. Lucy visited a doctor every other week, complaining of stomach aches. She exercised religiously, unless the stomach pain she regularly experienced became too severe. She was told that her fibroids were inflamed; other times she was treated for acid reflux, and most of the time, she was sent home and told to take Tums for indigestion. Lucy changed her diet and focused on eating healthy. Lucy's primary care doctor referred her to a gastroenterologist, who conducted what he considered to be the necessary tests. The doctor did not order a colonoscopy; he thought that Lucy, who was thirty years old, was too young to have colon cancer. Constant stomach pain became a part of Lucy's everyday life; she became an expert in tolerating and hiding her pain.

One evening, Shandra called Lucy and asked if they could go out for happy hour at the Staff NCO Club in Camp Pendleton. Shandra thought both she and Lucy needed a girls' night out to relax after a long week. They agreed they would go after 9:00 p.m., when the crowd was more interesting. They arrived at the club shortly after 10:00 p.m.; they stood next to the bar and ordered a drink. Lucy caught a glimpse of a short, dark-skinned gentleman seated at the bar. He wore a multicolored cardigan similar to what was known as a "nineties Bill Cosby sweater." The hem on his pants rose between the calf and ankle, exposing his long socks. He had a weary look and was staring at her butt.

Lucy, appalled, looked at the man directly and asked, "Why do you look like you've taken a bite of shit?"

Shandra burst out laughing, and the man smiled, exposing a gap in his bright white teeth. "I like what I'm looking at," he said.

"Don't you know it's rude to stare?" said Lucy.

"Let me buy you and your friend a drink," he replied. That was how Lucy met Nil.

Shortly after, he was deployed to Iraq. Their relationship developed long distance. Lucy sent him care packages, which he appreciated. Nil had been married twice and had two teenage children. In the beginning, Nil supported Lucy's effort to help pay school fees and feed several children in Kenya and even gave her a check for one thousand dollars; Lucy thought she had found an angel who understood her cause. When Nil returned to California, Lucy, now divorced from JV, moved in with Nil in his nearly empty apartment and brought living and bedroom furniture, serving dishes, art and collectibles, and everything else she had accumulated. Lucy had recently paid off her car, so she was happy that she owned her gold Honda CR-V with less than fifteen thousand miles on it.

On January 28, 2008, at 5:00 a.m. EST, Njeri received a call from a crying Lucy. *"Mwana witu niathie,"* she said, which translates, "Our child is gone."

Njeri did not see this coming. Shiku, their second-born sister, had been ill for a while. Recently, she had contacted pneumonia and was admitted to a hospital for long periods. Shiku was the responsible, go-getter sister who had set great examples to all. After leaving an unhappy relationship with the father of her children, she embarked on a journey of self-reliance and determination, focusing on raising her two teenage children, Julie and Koki. She had been doing great until she contracted pneumonia. Her death was a shock to the family and an unimaginable loss. The sisters spoke every day, and Shiku had insisted that Njeri, Lydiah, and Lucy not travel to see her until Easter so they could celebrate the Easter holidays. None of them could have predicted that they would not get that chance.

Both Lucy and Lydiah, who was living in upstate New York, could not make it to Shiku's funeral due to time and money. Lydiah flew to California to be with Lucy. During her visit, Lydiah witnessed an argument between Lucy and a drunk Nil that made her concerned about Lucy's well-being. Lucy asked Nil to be more respectful, especially in front of Lydiah. Nil's response was a string of insults that made Lucy so angry that she cried and then slapped him to make him stop; Nil punched her. The following morning, Nil acted as if nothing happened, and when Lydiah comforted him about hitting Lucy, he said he didn't remember.

A few months after Shiku's death, Nil received military orders to go Okinawa, Japan. Lucy called Njeri and told her they were going to the justice of peace in San Diego to get married. Njeri wanted to attend the ceremony, but Lucy said they could not wait for Njeri to get to California. Lucy promised to visit northern Virginia where Njeri and her family had settled after Tony's retirement from the military. In addition to Ethel, Njeri had a second daughter, Jazmine, who had been born shortly after they moved to New York.

Lucy and Nil visited Njeri in Virginia to celebrate Tony's birthday. Njeri thought that Nil seemed like a decent man. He was about twelve years older than Lucy. He did not talk much but offered to barbeque for the party. He stayed on the deck, drinking and barbequing, and Njeri noticed that he was beginning to loosen up. Before the party began, a drunk Nil started flirting with another woman who had come to the party. Lucy was embarrassed and convinced Nil to go back to the hotel. Lydiah and her husband Mike had traveled from New York for the party, and the sisters had a great time. A week later, Lucy and Nil left for Okinawa.

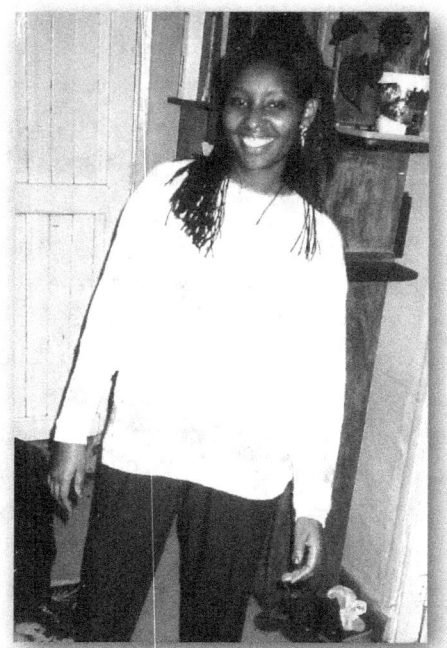

The last picture Lucy had of Shiku.

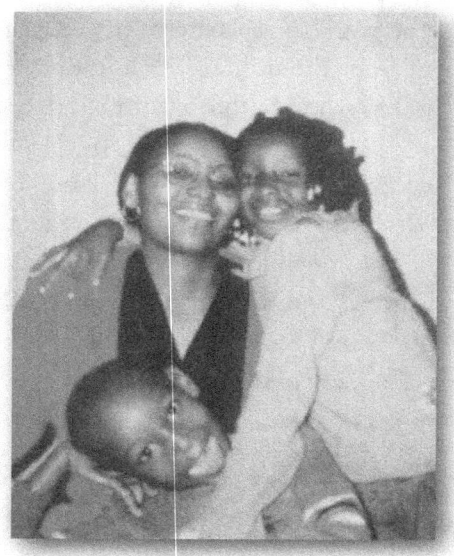

Shiku and her children Julie and Koki

CHAPTER 5

Short Tour of Okinawa

LUCY WAS EXCITED ABOUT GOING to Okinawa. She planned to find a job and save enough money to build Mami and Baba a dream house. She also planned on saving enough money to buy backpacks and school supplies for children in Kenya who could not afford them. When she arrived in Okinawa, she quickly realized that there was stiff competition among dependents for limited jobs at the military bases. It took a while to settle down. Lucy had sold her beloved Honda CR-V, which enabled her and Nil to get two used cars.

Nil no longer supported her sending money to family and those she helped. She felt uncomfortable going behind his back to send Mami any money. Worse, she had almost depleted her savings account after a few months without a job. Nil insisted that the money he made was his, and he was under no obligation to share. Lucy was bored staying at home, and after doing her housework several times over, she would watch the show *Farm Town*, which she was admittedly addicted to. She was ready to work at any available job.

Lucy soon found a part-time job, which kept her busy for a short while. The stomach issues were getting worse. One day she called Njeri and said she had had to pull over by the roadside because she could not drive due to the pain. The pain in the right side of her stomach was worse and more frequent. She thought the pain was caused by her inability to have regular bowel movements. One doctor explained that the reason she saw blood in her stool was due to internal hemorrhoids. The pain forced her to miss a few workdays; whenever she was well, Lucy soon formed her own circle of friends with whom she spent time. Lucy and Njeri called each other every other morning. Lucy confided that Nil had changed. Her infatuation phase with Nil was over. Lucy was not interested in going to nightclubs but did not mind that Nil enjoyed visiting them. She described him as moody, especially during the week.

"I think he is bipolar," she said. "One minute he is loving and the next he doesn't say a word for days. He always tries to make up by buying me gifts, and he has a new obsession with buying me Dooney and Bourke purses."

"Does he hit you?" Njeri was concerned.

"Hell no. He doesn't scare me. I would kick his ass. I think he has PTSD from his time in the Middle East. He doesn't sleep well. That is why he is moody."

"Stop making excuses for him. You know, you don't have to put up with bullshit; you have a place in Virginia. You are too far away."

"Don't worry. I won't be alone for too long. I found out that Shandra and James are coming to Okinawa for a few years. It will be nice to have people I think of as family around."

Njeri was relieved to hear that her old friends would be joining Lucy. She could trust them to be there for her little sister if she needed them. James and Shandra, accompanied by their teenage children Ashanti and Tre, arrived in Okinawa during the typhoon season; Lucy was happy. By this time, though, Lucy's stomach pains were more intense and left her debilitated. She spent most days in bed. However, the pain did not stop her from flying back to the United States to attend Lydiah's baby shower in New York.

Lucy was in a great mood when she met Njeri and Lydiah for the baby shower. She looked tired, and her eyes were bloodshot, but everyone assumed it was due to the travel. After the shower, Lucy wanted to rest because her stomach was cramping. She told her sisters that she had gone online to re-search why her bowel habits had changed. She was constipated often, and the stool was pencil thin. The search had brought up "symptoms of colon cancer." Lucy said she would suggest her doctor do a colonoscopy once she returned to Okinawa.

Lucy made her appointment early one morning. The doctor listened to her keenly but told her point-blank that it was very unlikely that she would get colon cancer.

"You are a thirty-four-year-old woman in good health," he said. "We did your blood work, and everything is fine. We can schedule a colonoscopy in two months."

Lucy left the office, feeling defeated. That afternoon, she called her supervisor, telling him she couldn't make it to work. She called Njeri to let her know that the pain was intolerable. "I don't know what else to do," Lucy said.

"What does Nil think?" Njeri asked.

"He doesn't think it's serious," Lucy responded. Lucy told Njeri that the last time she had a bowel movement, there had been blood in the stool. Njeri told Lucy go to the emergency room and not to leave unless they scheduled a colonoscopy.

The emergency room doctor took matters into his own hands. He called the chief surgeon, and before Lucy was discharged from the emergency room, a colonoscopy was scheduled two days later. Sure enough, a massive blockage the size of a grapefruit was in her colon. Because the doctors could not determine how serious Lucy's condition was, they scheduled surgery in a week. Lucy called her family to let them know she was all right and that she was hopeful that it was not cancer.

"They say that cancer doesn't hurt, but this pain hurts like hell, so I am sure it's not cancer," she joked.

The Sunday before surgery, Lucy went to church with one of her new friends. Lucy was sure that the message was meant for her. The pastor read from the Bible, the book of Matthew 6:25–34:

"Therefore I tell you, do not worry about your life, what you will eat or drink; or about your body, what you will wear. Is not life more than food and the body more than clothes? Look at the birds of the air; they do not sow or reap or store away in barns, and yet your heavenly Father feeds them. Are you not much more valuable than they? Can any one of you by worrying add a single hour to your life? "And why do you worry about clothes? See how the flowers of the field grow. They do not labor or spin. Yet I tell you that not even Solomon in all his splendor was dressed like one of these. If that is how God clothes the grass of the field, which is here today and tomorrow is thrown into the fire, will he not much more clothe you—you of little faith? So do not worry, saying, 'What shall we eat?' or 'What shall we drink?' or 'What shall we wear?' For the pagans run after all these things, and your heavenly Father knows that you need them. But seek first his kingdom and his righteousness, and all these things will be given to you as well. Therefore do not worry about tomorrow, for tomorrow will worry about itself. Each day has enough trouble of its own.

Lucy called Mami, Baba, and her siblings to let them know she was ready for the surgery and that she was at peace. Njeri called Shandra and Nil and asked that they keep her posted as to any development. They both promised to do so even though the time difference between Virginia and Okinawa was thirteen hours. Lucy was wheeled into the operating room in the early morning. The surgery was supposed to take three hours. Lucy was confident that this would be the end of the pain she had been feeling for a while. Little did she know that her world was about to change forever.

The surgery took eight hours to complete. Lucy's family was worried sick that they had not received any news. Mami kept calling Njeri because, even though she had spoken to Nil shortly before and after Lucy married him, communication was difficult as neither understood the other's English accent. At 3:30 a.m., Njeri's mobile phone rang; she could hear Shandra crying on the other line.

"Please tell me Lucy is OK," she told Shandra.

"Lucy is awake, but they think she has stage three or four colon cancer," Shandra responded.

Njeri felt sick to her stomach. She couldn't believe what she was hearing, Shandra wouldn't stop crying.

"Where is Nil?" She needed more information; she needed to know exactly what had happened. "Why hasn't Nil called? "Njeri asked. "Can you get him to call me please?"

"I will have him call you," Shandra responded. "I am sorry. I can't stop crying after seeing how extensive the surgery was. It is not fair to her." Shandra and Njeri continued to talk for a little while, but Njeri could not wrap her mind around what she was hearing. Finally, Shandra said, "Bye, I love you. I'll call you later."

Njeri responded, "I love you, too; I wish I was there, but I am not. Please, please, be there for her." Shandra promised she would.

Njeri could not go back to sleep. She called Mami and told her that Lucy had come through surgery and was too groggy to talk. Njeri decided not to mention the possibility of Lucy having colon cancer to Mami because she did not have enough information and frankly, she was hoping that Shandra was wrong and that Nil would call with the right information. Mami and Baba were relieved to hear the surgery went well. Njeri promised to call them back as soon as she heard from Nil.

Lucy woke up confused about her whereabouts. She had an uncomfortable feeling in her stomach, as though something was placed there. She reached at her belly and felt a bag. She tried to yank it out, but she couldn't. Lucy yelled for help; Nil was nearby. The doctors came in and explained to her that her condition was more serious than they had anticipated. They explained that they had had to remove half of her colon and a piece of her diaphragm and had given her a total hysterectomy. Lucy was too tired to comprehend, so she fell back asleep. Nil called Njeri, telling her that the doctors didn't know for sure what stage the cancer was in but they would do a biopsy.

The next time Lucy woke up, she knew she was in the intensive care unit. She saw someone walk in, sit next to her, stare for a few seconds, then walked away. She pressed the nurse button; indeed, the nurse explained that another patient had walked into her room unnoticed. The compression stockings for circulation were uncomfortable; Lucy asked the nurse if she could walk instead. The nurse was surprised, so she asked the doctor, who told her that if Lucy felt up to it, she could certainly walk. Lucy was aware that patients sometimes developed blood clots after surgery. Shandra walked into the room to find Lucy slowly walking using the IV stand to stabilize herself.

"You won't believe what your crazy sister is doing." Njeri could sense Shandra smiling at the end of the line. "She is walking."

It was almost midnight in Okinawa, which meant it was nearly 11:00 a.m. in Virginia when Lucy called Njeri. "I am OK, sis. I am not worried," she said. "The thing that was bothering me was removed, and I believe I am healed. Don't worry. I am not going anywhere. I have a lot of work to do."

Njeri knew Lucy would be OK. Lucy called Mami and Baba, assuring them that she was fine; they all believed her. A few days later, she was discharged from the hospital with a bag full of supplies and instructions on how to change the colostomy bag. Shandra, Nil's work colleagues, and Lucy's new friends in Okinawa visited and brought food and comfortable clothing to her while she was recuperating from surgery. Lucy appreciated their kindness and called her family to let them know she was in good hands. Lucy became comfortable changing the colostomy bag; however, Nil was the main caregiver, making sure that Lucy attempted to eat. He also became an expert on changing the colostomy bag, which Lucy had nicknamed "my friend."

A couple of weeks later, the doctors in Okinawa decided that Lucy had to return to the United States to get the treatment she needed. Since she and Nil had come from California, it was suggested that they return there or go to Hawaii where there were oncologists that could care for her. Lucy told Nil that she would like to move to Virginia to be close to her family. Nil thought it was a good idea, so he requested to have Lucy treated at the Walter Reed Army Medical Center in Washington, DC. Consultation appointments were scheduled. In September 2009, a year after Lucy had married Nil and moved to Okinawa, they made the long trip back to the United States through Los Angeles and arrived at the Reagan National Airport where Njeri couldn't wait to see her little sister again.

CHAPTER 6
It Could Be Worse

LUCY CALLED HER SISTER NJERI to say that they had missed their connection from the Los Angeles airport to Washington, DC. The trip went well for Lucy; Nil made sure she took her pain medication and helped change her colostomy bag as needed. She was tired but otherwise excited that she was going to see her sister. Lucy asked Njeri to make some Kenyan food that she could eat when she arrived. She also said that Nil had changed the plans for them to stay at Njeri's house, and instead, they would stay at the Mologne House, a hotel that housed wounded warriors and their families.

The flight arrived earlier than Njeri anticipated. Lucy and Nil were waiting at the arrival terminal when she pulled up. Lucy was wearing a sleeveless long, loose dress Njeri had sent her. She looked thinner, and her hair, which was braided, was in need of repair. Njeri jumped out of her car to hug her sister. Lucy held her sister tight and started crying uncontrollably. Njeri knew she had to be strong for her little sister; the only thing that came to mind was reciting the Lord's Prayer in their mother tongue; after the second line, Lucy joined in. Njeri thanked God for bringing Lucy back safely, and after the prayer, they were both smiling. Nil gave Njeri a hug and began loading the suitcases in the car. He had rented a vehicle, so he asked if Njeri could take him to the rental place.

Getting to Walter Reed took a long time. Njeri was using an old GPS, and Nil was following. She kept taking wrong turns. Eventually, Nil asked that Njeri follow, and they reached the Mologne House at around 9:00 p.m. The room they would be staying in had a microwave, a refrigerator, and a nice-size shower. They also had a living room area for guests. Njeri brought in a small cooler with food Lucy had requested. She washed a plate and placed on it a small amount of food to heat up in the microwave. Lucy took two bites and pushed the food away.

"She is not eating, she needs her strength so, she needs to eat more," Nil said.

Lucy looked sadly at her sister and said, "Sis, it's not that I don't want to eat. I can't eat. The food tastes weird. As soon as I eat, the food comes out of the colostomy bag, which grosses me out. I just need to take a shower and go to sleep; tomorrow I'll feel better."

Nil removed a box of Saran Wrap and set out the supplies Lucy needed to change the colostomy bag. Lucy explained that she had to tie the plastic wrap around her stomach to make sure the area stayed dry while she took the shower. Njeri helped Lucy wrap the plastic and turned the water on for Lucy's shower. Afterward, Lucy lay flat on the bed. Nil was waiting to help Lucy change the bag.

Lucy smiled at her sister and joked, "He takes this very seriously. He does it with precision, and I am not supposed to interrupt him when he is doing it."

Nil lined up the measuring guide, adhesive remover, skin protector, wafer, pencil, stomach adhesive paste, new pouch, scissors, and a washcloth. He removed the used pouch, wiped the surrounding area, and patted it dry. Next, Nil marked the stoma, marked the wafer, and cut the hole and applied skin protector where he would place the wafer. He snapped the new pouch onto the wafer and pulled it a little to make sure it was OK. Nil completed the process without saying a word. Lucy dressed in her pajamas and said she was ready to lie down. It was now midnight, and Njeri needed to make her way back to Virginia because she was coming back to the Mologne House the following day.

Njeri slept for three hours, and then it was time to go to work. She arrived on time and sent an e-mail to her supervisor, Pam, asking for a meeting. Her supervisor told her she was free, so Njeri walked into the office and sat down. She explained that her sister had arrived from Japan and needed help. She asked to take time off but didn't know how much time. She knew she would be accompanying her sister to appointments, but they were not scheduled yet. Njeri's supervisor agreed to let her telecommute when she could; otherwise she had enough leave if she needed to be away for a longer period.

That afternoon, Njeri arrived at Mologne House to find Lucy waiting for her. Lucy hugged her tightly. She seemed well rested and had more energy. Lucy explained that Nil had gone to the store to buy snacks. Lucy said they had ventured out around the neighborhood, but she had gotten tired and come back to rest. Lucy continued talking about her morning.

"The bag was leaking, so I woke up to change it at four in the morning. I didn't want to wake Nil who was sleeping soundly, so I did it myself. I've become quite good actually. Looking at the bag used to make me sad, but I realize the bag is helping me remove waste from my body until I am healed. I now see it as a friend.

"I couldn't fall asleep after changing the bag, so I started thinking. I thought about how lucky I am that I have this option. I can only imagine what happens to people around the world when they have a mass in their colon; most likely they are not treated. In the end they just die, their families not knowing what killed them. I am so grateful to God that I have people that love and care about me. I am grateful for Nil because he has been there for me; I was surprised because I did not think he was capable of handling it. He loves me in his own way.

"I lay in bed, thinking how I have to fight to get better. They are telling me it's advanced cancer, either stage three or four. They don't know yet, but we will know soon. I am only thirty-four years old. I had a lot of dreams, one of which was to have children. I wanted to build Mami a nice house. I wanted to travel the world. I wanted to help my family and others. I now know for sure that I will never have children of my own, and I am OK with that. I have always considered my nieces and nephews as my own children.

"I cannot give up on my dreams; there are many ways I can help children without being a parent. I don't believe God is so cruel to let my dreams die. I know the road ahead is tough, but I know God is with me. I know he has a plan for me and that I am already healed.

"This morning when daylight came, I got out of bed, grabbed my clothes, and changed in the bathroom so I did not wake Nil. I grabbed the keys and walked out of the room to the elevator. As I was waiting, I was joined by an older couple who were wheeling a young man who I assume was their son. The young man did not have hands or legs. It was his torso on the wheelchair. I am sure those parents still thought of him as their son. We were joined by other amputees, and we all got into the elevator. I later realized they were going to have breakfast at the cafeteria downstairs. These young men are wounded warriors. They have been shot at, had their body parts blown up, but they are still here. They have survived painful experiences, more than any of us would ever understand. If they can move on, so can I. All I know is that things could be a lot worse. So, I will not feel sorry for myself. I will not ask why me. In fact, why not me? We are all God's children going through life experiences.

"I thought, These soldiers had dreams before they were wounded, and I am sure they have dreams now. The only difference is that the dreams have changed. My dreams will have to change, too, but I will never give up. I have to be strong for Mami and the rest of you. I have to carry on. This is just a temporary roadblock on my journey. I don't want anyone feeling sorry for me or treating me any different. I am still me, only with a new friend and an illness that will be cured. As a matter of fact, I know I will live to see my nine-tieth birthday. I sometimes have a pity party, but all I have to do is remember it could be a lot worse."

"Amen," was Njeri's response.

CHAPTER 7

Diagnosis

FOR THE FIRST APPOINTMENT AT Walter Reed, Njeri accompanied Lucy. Nil could not join them because he had to report to the Quantico Marine Corps Base where he was being transferred. At the primary care clinic, they checked in with the receptionist. A few minutes later, a nurse called Lucy's name, recorded her weight and blood pressure, then escorted them to a small room.

A young doctor wearing khaki pants and a long white coat walked in and shook both their hands. "My name is Dr. Rogers; I am one of the resident doctors here. I will be asking you about your history, which I will relay to my boss. He will come in and talk to you afterward. So, tell me what brings you here?"

Lucy told Dr. Rogers her story, starting with when she started getting severe stomach pains and ending with how she ended up in the emergency room. Dr. Rogers took notes as Lucy spoke; he asked for clarification when he needed to. After he received answers to his questions, he said he would return with his boss.

Lucy and Njeri were left in the room for what seemed like a long time. They passed the time by talking about conversations with Mami, Baba, their sister Lydiah, who was now a mother, and their sister Gloria who was planning on migrating to the United States. They talked about their sister Nancy and brother Jeff, who they missed dearly, and all the nephews and nieces. They were deep in conversation when the door opened.

Dr. Rogers came in and shook both of their hands again, saying, "My name is Dr. Rogers. I am one of the resident doctors here. I will be asking you about your history, which I will relay to my boss. He will come in and talk to you afterward. So, tell me what brings you here?"

Lucy and Njeri looked at each other and burst out laughing. Dr. Rogers looked confused; Lucy spoke first. "Dr. Rogers, are you that tired? We already spoke to you, but I could repeat if you want me to."

Dr. Rogers's face turned red with embarrassment. "I am so sorry," he said. "I am going to sleep soon; it's been a long night."

Dr. Rogers returned with two other physicians who wore military uniforms. The older physician jumped straight to the point. "Your pathology results are in, and I am sorry to tell you that you have stage four colon cancer."

The room fell silent for a few seconds. Lucy asked, "What does this mean in terms of treatment?"

The doctor explained that Walter Reed would coordinate Lucy's care with Georgetown University and the National Institutes of Health (NIH). He told them that he had appointments to meet with the oncologist, Dr. Delmas, who would be her primary oncologist and caregiver scheduled for the next day. Two days later, Lucy was expected at Georgetown University Lombardi Comprehensive Cancer Center. The military insurance, TriCare, had set up all these appointments.

Lucy was asked if she had any questions, and she said, "Am I allowed to make love with my husband? He wanted to know."

The doctor's reply was, "If you want to." Lucy laughed loudly, and everyone in the room followed.

Njeri, Nil, and Lucy arrived early the following morning to meet with the oncologist. Dr. Delmas greeted them warmly. He explained in detail Lucy's condition and that it was difficult to tell where the cancer originated. He told Lucy that she had a long battle ahead of her and it was important to have a good support system. He explained that she had the option of receiving chemo at Walter Reed or Georgetown. Dr. Delmas recommended genetic testing for the family and said that most insurance companies did not cover the cost. Nil asked Dr. Delmas how long he thought Lucy might live. Dr. Delmas responded by saying that every patient was different.

For the Georgetown appointment, family friend Diane, who worked as a registered nurse, joined Njeri and Nil. They were escorted to a small room with two chairs. Lucy sat on the medical exam table, Njeri and Diane sat on the chairs and Nil stood beside Lucy. The doctor walked in and introduced himself as Dr. Lee. He repeated most of what Dr. Delmas had told them.

"How much time does Lucy have?" Nil asked abruptly.

"That's hard to say, every cancer patient is different," Dr. Lee responded.

"Working here as a doctor, I am sure you've seen patients in Lucy's condition. On average, how long do they normally last?" Nil insisted.

"Most likely, the disease will end her life. However, there are clinical trials that work for some patients. There is no telling exactly how much her life will be extended."

"Treatment will work for Lucy," Njeri jumped in.

"What if the treatment doesn't work?" Njeri and Diane looked at Nil with disapproval. Lucy stared at the wall without saying a word.

"If the treatment does not work, Lucy has two years at most," Dr. Lee finally answered Nils's question. Lucy checked out at that point. Her face looked like she had seen a ghost. She did not hear anything else the doctor said after that. He said the cancer had metastasized to different parts of the body, so it would be difficult to treat with existing medications. However, he offered Lucy an opportunity to join a case study with a new medication. Lucy was thrilled at the opportunity of being offered a new drug. Before leaving, the nurse said she would get in touch after making the arrangements and getting authorization from Tricare.

No one said a word during the ride back to the Mologne House. Lucy's face was soaked with tears, and she slowly wiped them and sniffed. Njeri and Diane were in shock. Nil concentrated on driving. As soon as they walked through the door, Njeri could no longer hold her tears, and together, the two sisters cried uncontrollably.

Lucy was the first one to speak. "Only God knows when someone will die. I will not die within two years."

They stared at each other and simultaneously did what they had done as children when things got tough: they recited the Lord's Prayer as Mami had taught them as children.

Ithe witu uri iguru (Our father in heaven)
Ritwa riaku riamurwo (May your name be revered)
Uthamaki waku uke (May your kingdom come)
Ta uria wendete we (As you would want it to be)
Niwikaga guku thi (You do on earth)
Ta uria wikugu kuu iguru (As you do in heaven)
Tuhe umuthi irio cia gutuigana (Give us enough food for today)
Na utwohere mehia maitu (And forgive us our sins)
Utauria twohagira aria matwihagiria (As we forgive those who sin against us)
Na ndugatutwari magerioni (Do not lead us into temptation)
No gutuhonikia uruini (But save us from evil)
Ni undu uthamaki ni waku (For the kingdom is yours)
Ona hinya, ona kugocuo (And the power and glory)
Tene na tene, Amen (Forever and ever, Amen).

When they were done, they hugged again and wiped their tears. Njeri went into the refrigerator, found some leftovers, and warmed them for Lucy, who took only a couple of bites and then said she wanted to rest.

For two weeks, Lucy did not hear back from Georgetown. Njeri contacted the nurse, asking for an update. The nurse responded that the insurance was taking a long time to authorize treatment at Georgetown. Lucy did not want to deal with the hassle of waiting for the insurance authorizations. She made the decision to get her chemotherapy treatment at Walter Reed and have Dr. Delmas as her oncologist.

"I liked him when we met. I have a good feeling about him," she said.

CHAPTER 8

First Round of Treatment

Lucy arrived at the Walter Reed Army Medical Center Oncology and Hematology department early on a Tuesday morning. Dr. Delmas and his team were waiting. Dr. Delmas explained that the treatment would be aggressive because the cancer had metastasized. Lucy would require ten rounds of chemotherapy, given every other week. Every other Wednesday, Lucy would have a standing appointment to get a combination of drugs including Avastin, 5-FU, Oxalipalatin, and Leucovorin infused for that day. Before leaving, she would get a pump for slower infusion for Wednesday night, all day Thursday, and half of Friday. She was expected to return the pump to the hospital on Fridays. To reduce the number of sticks, Lucy was scheduled to receive an implantable port on the upper left arm the next day.

The surgery to implant the port took a couple of hours under moderate anesthesia. Njeri and Nil were waiting for Lucy when she was done. "I could hear everything they were doing, and I tried to talk but couldn't. I actually felt some pain," Lucy said. "I am glad that is over, though. No pain compares to what I was feeling before surgery." They went back to Mologne House for lunch. Lucy ate a couple of French fries and said she couldn't stand the smell of food. She decided to rest for the afternoon. In a week's time, chemo treatment would begin.

By the time Wednesday arrived, Lucy was extremely anxious about starting chemo. A few days prior, the nurses had drawn her blood, and the results indicated that treatment could move forward. Lucy was put in a private room. The infusion started at 8:00 a.m. and did not end until 4:00 p.m. In between, different professionals visited Lucy, and each extended an offer to help and to answer any questions.

The psychologist asked, "Would you prefer to speak privately, or can your sister and husband stay?" Lucy said that they could stay. The psychologist wanted to hear what Lucy's thoughts on having cancer were. "I am not angry. I get sad once in a while but not for long. I remind myself how lucky I am. I am getting good care. I am surrounded by people who love me, and I believe that everything will be fine. I have a lot to look forward to and can't wait for the next chapter in my life. I don't worry too much about it," she said.

Next was the dietician, who offered advice on what to eat in order to make sure her body would receive proper nutrients during chemo. The dietician went straight to the point. "Most likely, your appetite will decrease after chemo, and food will have a metallic taste and probably will smell bad to you. It's important to maintain proper nutrition, as it will aid in your healing. Eat regularly. The doctor said you are not on any diet restriction. The most important thing to remember is chew, chew, and chew your food."

"That sounds tedious," Lucy responded. "How long should I chew?"

"If not sure, count to forty or even fifty," said the dietician.

The chaplain came in next and asked if Lucy had any religious preference, to which Lucy responded, "I am a born-again Christian. I believe in the Bible promises. I believe that no matter what I am experiencing, God is with me, and he will not abandon me." This opened the conversation for the chaplain, who began talking about the book of Job, the faithful servant of God, and how he was tested. The chaplain talked to Lucy for almost an hour.

Before he left, he asked Lucy, "What if it's not God's plan for you to remain on this earth but to be with him in his kingdom?"

"I hope his plan is not for me to join him right now," Lucy responded with a giggle. "I have some work to do. But if it's his will, oh well; no one will live forever. Each one of us will leave this world the same way, by dying."

After the day-long infusion, the pharmacist brought the pump, strapped it around Lucy, and set it to infuse for three days. Before leaving, Lucy received instructions to avoid crowds, young children, and sick people because chemotherapy treatment weakens the immune system. She was told to drink a lot of water and to flush the toilet twice after using because the medicine she would be taking was very toxic. She was also told that her extremities would be sensitive to cold. She was given emergency numbers to call in case her body temperature rose above one hundred degrees.

That first night Lucy felt a burst of energy. She did not sleep at all. She wondered what to do, but all she could think of was to unpack her clothes and repack them. It was a very long night, and Lucy decided to come up with creative ways to spend her time while undergoing chemo; this began a creativity phase that lasted until the day she died. She knew she had to continue helping the children in Kenya. She also knew it would be a while before she found a new job. She remembered how she made chapati for Mami to sell for extra income as a young girl in order to help others. She made a decision to try different projects in order to generate income. Jewelry making seemed like a great idea.

The Friday after she returned the pump was a different story. Lucy could barely walk because of exhaustion. She spent most of the time sleeping, and Nil and Njeri had to remind her to at least drink and eat. Lucy had never felt that tired before and could not explain the extent of the fatigue. It took five days for her to return to her new normal.

Before the second round of chemo, Nil made plans to return to Okinawa. They had left due to the medical emergency, and he had not checked out of his duty station. The military required him to check out of his previous station before checking into Quantico. Njeri prepared a room in her house for Lucy. Nil and Lucy checked out of Mologne House, and Nil flew to Okinawa for two weeks. Plans were also made to have Mami visit the United States from Kenya.

For the second round of chemo, Njeri drove Lucy from Virginia to Walter Reed and arrived before 6:00 a.m. After her vitals were taken and it was confirmed that Lucy was strong enough for chemo, the infusions began. Njeri made sure that Lucy was settled, and then she drove the forty miles back to Virginia to get her uncle Warui, who had stopped by to visit Lucy; he was traveling back to Atlanta that morning. Lucy had not seen Uncle Warui (who lived in Kenya) since immigrating to the United States. She was happy that their uncle stopped by to see her before returning to Kenya. Uncle Warui had come to Atlanta to wrap up things after his daughter Martha suddenly passed away. At Dulles airport, Njeri got permission to escort her uncle to the gate; after he boarded, Njeri headed back to the hospital.

Mami's plane was due to arrive at 5:00 p.m., but despite leaving early for Dulles airport, Njeri got caught in the rush hour. Njeri had no way of communicating that she would be late since Mami's Kenya mobile phone did not work in the United States. Just as she arrived at the airport, Njeri's phone rang. It was Mami; she had made some friends who allowed her to use their phone to call Njeri. Despite the long journey, Mami said she was not too tired and was anxious to see Lucy.

Njeri spotted Mami from a distance; she was wearing a long, flowing dress and a brown cardigan. Mami was smiling as she spoke to a young lady and a gentleman that were standing beside her. Njeri ran to hug Mami, who held her tightly and quickly introduced her new friends.

"This is my firstborn, Njeri, and these are the nice people who let me borrow their phone. I saw them on the plane all the way from Nairobi, through Amsterdam to here, so I felt like I knew them. They speak Swahili. I was telling them about Lucy and how she loves bananas. I had cut down the hanging cluster and had a bunch of bananas, but the customs people would not let me bring them in."

"Mami, I told you not to bring any raw fruit or vegetables. It is not allowed," Njeri said. "Furthermore, you can get all that here."

Mami looked at Njeri as though she didn't know what she was saying. "It does not taste the same. Nothing tastes the same. Those bananas were from my farm, and I am told they have the best taste. Oh well, I hope they enjoy them because I know they will not throw them away," Mami said.

Njeri decided to discontinue the banana conversation and said, "Lucy will be done shortly, so let's get on the road, Mami. Thank you for waiting with her." Mami invited her new friends to visit her at her farm for bananas when they returned to Kenya.

Lucy had completed the infusions and had been given the take-home pump when Njeri arrived back at Walter Reed. Mami walked hurriedly in front of Njeri and ran to Lucy when she saw her. Tears of joy streamed down Lucy's face, and she could barely speak due to laryngeal dysesthesia where her voice had changed and she said it felt as if her throat was closing. Mami started singing and giving praises to God for allowing her to see her child. Mami would not let Lucy's hand go and was not in a hurry to leave the hospital. She thanked the nurses in Swahili, not caring whether they understood or not, and then they started on the long journey back to Virginia.

During this round of chemo, Lucy experienced mild peripheral neuropathy, which left her hands and feet feeling numb. After the third day, Lucy suffered extreme fatigue and spent the next few days in and out of consciousness. Njeri took time off from work in order to help change the colostomy bag. Mami prepared different foods for Lucy, and for the first time since the diagnosis, Lucy enjoyed eating small amounts of food. Mami had the patience to feed Lucy ten times a day if that was what it took for her to finish a small plate of food. Lydiah and her family visited as often as they could. Nil called every day to check how things were going. It was a few days before Thanksgiving, and the family had a lot to be grateful for.

Nil returned two days before Thanksgiving. The house they would be moving into in Quantico would be ready just before Christmas, so he rented a suite at the Quantico Crossroads.

"Where is my wife?" Nil yelled as he walked through the door. Lucy was sitting at the kitchen table, eating dinner.

"She is right here," she answered. They left Njeri's house that evening.

On Thanksgiving morning, Lucy went to Walter Reed to get her blood drawn in preparation for the next round of chemo. The vice president of the United States, Joseph Biden, was visiting wounded warriors at Walter Reed Hospital. Lucy met him, took a picture on her phone, and could not wait to return to Njeri's house to show the picture. Although the quality of the picture was not particularly good, it made Lucy's day. Thanksgiving Day of 2009 was a great family day. The feast included American and Kenyan food made by Mami. That day, Lucy ate more than she had eaten in several months.

There was no question that Mami was going to move in with Lucy once they settled into the new house; the main purpose of her visit was to take care of her child. Nil and Lucy's new house had three bedrooms, and Mami settled into a guest bedroom. She woke up every morning to prepare Lucy's food. She cooked what she knew, Kenyan food, for her and Nil. Soon, it became clear that Nil was not fond of this new arrangement. He complained about Mami's cooking and Lucy's family always being at the house. It was uncomfortable for Mami, so she asked Njeri to pick her up on weekends so she could prepare Lucy's food at Njeri's house. Nil tried to make Lucy eat the food he cooked, but she had a hard time digesting meat, his preferred dish.

A few days after her third round of chemo, Lucy developed a fever and had to be rushed to the hospital. She was admitted for several days, and Mami returned to Njeri's house. After Lucy's discharge, Mami returned to living with Lucy and continued to take care of her. Mami had brought some beads from Kenya and started teaching Lucy how to make necklaces. It became their pastime. Mami stayed in her room most of the time but would not leave Lucy; Nil barely spoke to her, which made Mami more uncomfortable and Lucy embarrassed. For both Christmas and New Year's, Lucy's family visited to cheer her up, as she was too tired to go to Njeri's. There was no mistaking that Nil was getting irritated each time the family came over. Eventually, Lucy wrote Nil's older brother, asking to talk to him, but there was no response. By this time, it was no secret that the family was not welcome to visit with Lucy.

By the third round of chemo, Lucy's hair had begun to fall out. First, she cut it short and brushed it back, but eventually, she asked Nil to shave it off. As Nil prepared the tools to shave her head, Lucy looked at both Mami and Njeri with tears in her eyes and said, "It is funny how things change. Less than two years ago, I was asked to pause for a photo shoot by my hairdresser to showcase how stylish my hair was. Today, the hair which I valued and saw as part of me is gone. I've been trying to hold on to it because it felt like I was losing a part of me. However, I recognize it's just hair, and it will grow back someday." Njeri and Mami couldn't agree more.

By March, Mami decided it was time to move out of Nil and Lucy's house and only to visit for the three days when Lucy was exhausted after chemo.

The treatment had become routine for the family. Everything was planned around Lucy's chemo, whether it was visiting with friends, work schedules, sightseeing for Mami, everything. Mami, Njeri, Lydiah, and other family and friends stayed away from Lucy and Nil's house and only visited when Lucy was unable to come to them. At this time, Lucy had to share the one car Nil owned, which made her mad, knowing she used to have her own. Sometimes Nil would refuse to let her use the car. Lucy took her hobby of making jewelry very seriously. Each day, when not extremely fatigued from chemo, she dragged her big white storage container from the closet to the living room. In it, she kept her black beading mat, multi colored beads, chain and round nose pliers, wire and wire cutters, clasps, stoppers and other items. She moved her coffee table out of the way to set up a work area and sat on the floor. Her designs were contemporary necklaces, earrings and bracelets based on jewelry traditionally worn by Kenyan women. She and Mami spent hours perfecting a design by doing it over until they were satisfied. They chatted about everything for many hours while working on their craft. Njeri sold the jewelry fast enough for Lucy to buy materials to make more. The profit Lucy made was sent to Kenya to help "her" children.

"I know you guys don't like to come to the house, but remember, it's my house, too, Mami," Lucy said one afternoon as they were making the necklaces. "I will talk to him."

"Don't say anything to him. It will make him mad. I came here for you, and I will not leave until you are better, so don't worry, Lucy. I have thick skin, so Nil will not deter me from seeing you. He doesn't understand that we are not here to take his place. Our people and his people are from different cultures. Tony has been to Kenya, so he understands that we are not beggars as they show on television."

Njeri felt the need to intervene. "Mami, it's not everyone. I have lived in the United States for a long time, and people are either good or bad. Nil has only been married to Lucy for a year and wants her all to himself. He thinks we are interfering with his relationship."

Mami jumped in before Njeri finished what she was saying. "He should ask himself why until now none of us have seen him. He should understand that family must come together when one of them needs help. He acts like we want something from him when the truth is, we want nothing from him. Anyway, he will not stop me from being with my child; Lucy will be well soon, and I will go back to my home."

Lucy laughed and said, "He is lucky we are not in Kenya. Can you imagine how many people would be showing up at the house on a daily basis to see me?" They all laughed.

Mami added, "When Shiku was in the hospital, the nurses had to beg people to leave. When they asked for blood donations, so many people showed up they had to turn them away. This is what families and friends are about. Nothing is bigger than showing love toward others."

Mami left shortly after Lucy's ninth round of chemo and the MRI that showed that the cancer cells had disappeared. Gloria arrived from Kenya a few days before Mami left to ensure that Lucy would always have someone around. Soon, it was time for Lucy's tenth round of chemo; she declared it would be the final one, ever. She was looking forward to completing this tedious, exhausting, but necessary process.

It was a rainy spring morning when Njeri and Gloria took Lucy to get that final round of chemo. The traffic was slow on I-95 from Virginia, which was typical when there was inclement weather. The outside conditions did not seem to affect Lucy in the least. She was happy and excited that she would no longer have chemo; she was looking forward to the colostomy reversal, which the doctors told her would be done after she completed chemo treatment. She was looking forward to returning to work. To Lucy, this was the break she has been waiting for, and nothing could bring her down.

The tenth round of infusion began shortly after Lucy arrived at the hospital. The psychiatrist, the chaplain, and the dietician stopped by as they usually did, but this time with smiles and well wishes.

Right before the conclusion of the process at 3:30 p.m., Dr. Delmas stopped by and gave Lucy a big hug. "I am so glad how things turned out, Lucy. The drugs have worked well, so we will use the same treatment if the cancer comes back," he said.

"Dr. Delmas, the cancer is not coming back so don't worry about it," Lucy responded.

"I hope so, Lucy; the fact that you have no cancer cells in your body is a miracle. You have maintained a positive attitude throughout, and I am so proud of you. Just remember that if you maintain this positive attitude, you have already won half the cancer battle," Dr. Delmas said.

After the pump that Lucy would take home for the slow infusion was connected, the nurses gave Lucy a bell that was reserved for patients who complete chemo treatment. She rose from her chair, placed the bell on the table, and with a huge smile on her face, slapped her hand hard on the ringer. The bell rang very loudly followed by cheering and clapping in the entire chemo section.

The nurses burst out singing Ray Charles's song. *"Hit the road, Jack, and don't you come back no more, no more, no more, no more. Hit the road, Jack, and don't you come back no more. What you say? Hit the road, Jack, and don't you come back no more, no more, no more, no more. Hit the road, Jack, and don't you come back no more."*

Lucy's joy could not be contained; her smile said it all.

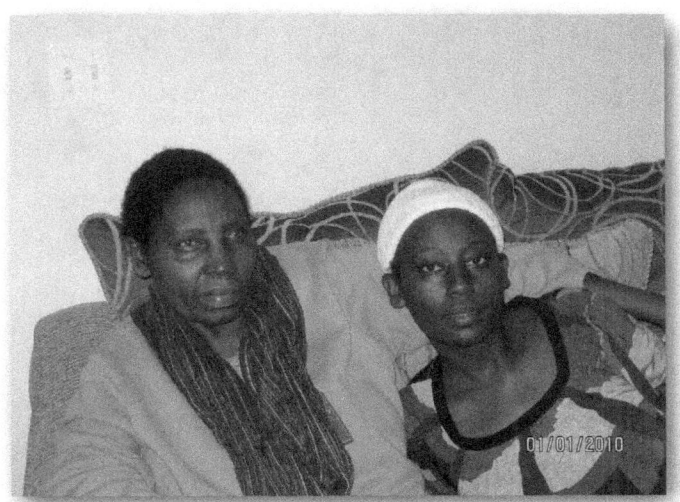

Lucy and Mami in Virginia 2010

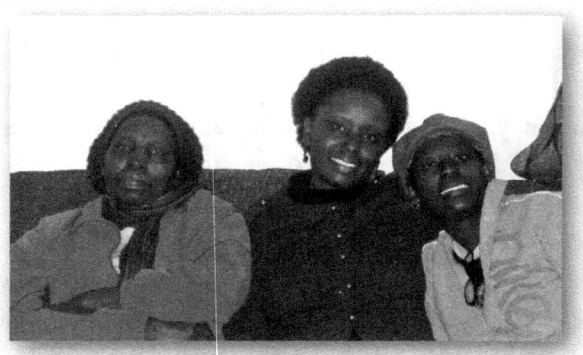

Njeri visiting Lucy and Mami

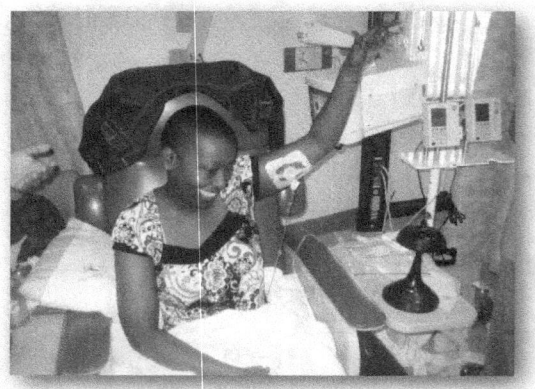

Lucy ringing the bell at the end of the first round of chemo treatment

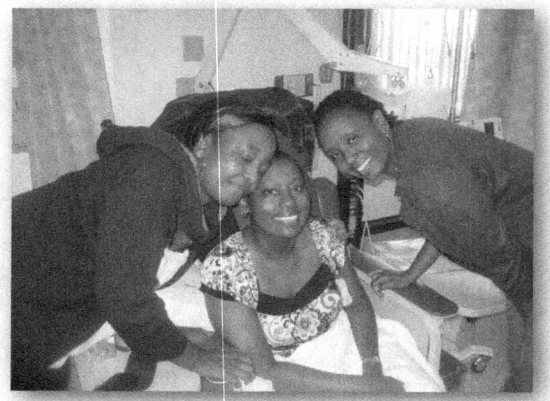

Gloria and Njeri on the day Lucy completed the first round of chemo.

CHAPTER 9

Remission

AFTER THE TENTH ROUND OF chemo, Lucy recovered faster from the fatigue than during the previous rounds. She had a new lease on life and couldn't wait to write her next chapter. She made a promise to herself that when the chemo stopped, she would resume her life with gusto. On the first Monday after chemo, Lucy drove to Wal-Mart and bought a twenty-four-by-thirty-six-inch poster board. She created a new vision board; her priorities were now different, and she wanted to be reminded of them every day.

Lucy's vision board included pictures of a house, representing the one she would build for Mami and Baba; dollar bills representing financial success from her business; a picture of school supplies representing her goal to support children with education; a blue ribbon showing her commitment to help search for colon cancer cure; airplanes and hotels representing her desire to travel; and a Bible representing her faith and trust in God. She still had mild peripheral neuropathy on her fingers and toes, and her nails, hands, and feet were black from the side effects of chemo. Her hair grew back soft and curly, and Lucy joked that African American women who were getting curly perms were in essence going after the chemo hair look without knowing it.

Dr. Delmas, the oncologist, asked Lucy to return to Walter Reed in three months for a consultation with gastroenterologist surgeons to explore the possibility having the colostomy reversed. Lucy looked forward to this appointment. In the meantime, she was ready to live her life doing the things she loved, including spending time with her family whenever she could, but she did not have a car.

Nil used their car to go back and forth to work, so Lucy volunteered to drop him off at work so she could have the car during the day, but he refused. Lucy needed to get around, so she asked Njeri to take her to buy her own car. She liked the Toyota Corolla because she could afford the monthly payments based on her income selling the Kenyan jewelry. Despite Lucy's FICO score of 780 and the salesman's eagerness to sell the car, Lucy didn't have proof of employment.

"Do you have someone who can cosign the loan for you?" the salesman asked. Njeri said she could.

"Actually, I don't want my sister to commit to this without giving it careful thought," Lucy responded. "I know my husband will cosign the loan as long as he doesn't have to pay for it. I will come back another day, but save that Corolla for me."

Njeri and Lucy left the dealership and decided to have lunch at Panera Bread. Lucy was upset that she couldn't get a car on her own, and she couldn't let it go. "All my adult life, I have strived to be financially independent and hate begging for anything. When I needed extra money, I took on a second job. Before going to Okinawa, Nil convinced me to sell my car so we could buy two used cars for use while posted there. Now he won't even let me use his car. Recently, his favorite phrase is my 'my money,' 'my car,' 'my house,' 'my laptop.' I am getting sick of it. Can you believe he called me lazy the other day and said I need to find a job?" Lucy vented.

"Why would he say that to you?" Njeri was getting angry. "What is really going on, sis?"

"Njeri, stop worrying. I can take care of myself, and there is nothing going on other than his mood swings."

"Well, I think it's best if we stop coming over to your house. I am sure he wants to spend more time doing fun things with you now that you are not getting chemo."

"Oh, please," Lucy responded. "The only thing he considers fun is going to the nightclubs, dancing with people half his age, and I am not doing that. The week after my chemo, I asked him to go to the movies. He said that theaters smell like urinals." She laughed out loud. "I don't allow him to get into my head because I know who I am, and being lazy I am not. Whenever he feels guilty after treating me wrong, he goes to the Marine Corps Exchange and buys me something, mostly a Dooney and Bourke handbag, then apologizes. I know he loves me, but he has been through terrible relationships with women and thinks every woman is after his money."

"You are a grown woman. I learned years ago not to interfere with your relationship with any man, but be careful, sis. His behavior toward you could become worse. First, he doesn't want your family at your house, and now he is becoming possessive materially. To me, this is classic abuser behavior."

After lunch, Njeri took Lucy to the house she shared with Nil at Quantico Marine Corps base. Lucy asked Njeri to come in for some Kenyan chai. Nil was still at work so Njeri obliged. They continued talking while Lucy was making the tea, which was a process; first, she boiled the water, adding loose Kenya tea and spices. After the water boiled, Lucy added milk. She brought the tea to the table and together, they enjoyed the chai as they had for many years. Nil walked in as Njeri was finishing the cup of tea; he went upstairs without saying a word. Njeri left the house, shaking her head, wondering if there was a problem between them. Two days later, Nil drove to the dealership with Lucy and decided that the Toyota Corolla Lucy had picked would have his name only. He, however, made it very clear to Lucy that she was responsible for the monthly payments.

Lucy finally had her freedom; she could come and go as she pleased but always made sure she was home before Nil returned from work. She carried her colostomy supplies and could change the pouch standing up.

Lucy discovered where crafts shops were in northern Virginia and found different charms and beads for her jewelry. Njeri had been selling the jewelry to her work friends; her biggest client was Donna Marie, who later became Lucy's friend. Word of Lucy's fine jewelry spread among friends who purchased it, enabling Lucy to finance her own business without asking Nil for money. Lucy was making enough money to pay for her car and provide school supplies and food for the children in Kenya. She needed to grow her business, so she created a website through Etsy and announced that some of the profit would go toward colon cancer research. Lucy's friend, Linda, whom she met while working in California, introduced her to glass beads that made bracelets that rivaled PANDORA, the famous jewelry makers. Lucy couldn't have been happier.

Three months after chemo, Lucy asked Njeri if she could accompany her and Nil to Walter Reed for a consultation to see if the colostomy could be reversed. The surgeon assured Lucy that she was a possible candidate, as she had recuperated well after chemo. His main concern was that there could be tissue buildup that would make it impossible to reverse the procedure, which meant that Lucy would spend the rest of her life using a colostomy bag.

"I will not have that problem," Lucy confidently told the surgeon.

One early morning during the third week of June in 2010, Lucy was admitted to Walter Reed hospital to have the colostomy reversal surgery. Njeri and Gloria were in the waiting room when Lucy and Nil arrived. Lucy was happy to see them and joked, "When I leave the hospital, I will be walking around, farting all over the place just to annoy people." They burst out laughing. "People take passing gas and pooping for granted, but it's almost ten months since I had that experience, and I can't wait to do it." She was serious.

The surgery was scheduled for 8:00 a.m. However, more serious cases of wounded soldiers being brought in for operations kept bumping the surgery. Lucy patiently waited. At noon, the surgeon came over to the room where Lucy was waiting and asked to speak to her privately. Gloria and Njeri left the room and waited at the reception area. After fifteen minutes, the nurse asked Gloria and Njeri to come back to the room. Lucy was crying, and Nil looked like he had cried, too.

"The surgeon thinks I have too much scar tissue, so he is suggesting that I skip the surgery. He says he is not so sure that it will be a success and I might wake up still wearing a colostomy bag. I told him I will take that chance."

At 2:00 p.m., Lucy was wheeled to the operating room. Njeri and Gloria went to the library to wait for the news. Nil had booked a room at Mologne House and surprised the sisters when he asked if they would like to wait in the room instead of the library. They had left the house at 4:00 a.m., so they were happy that he offered. At 6:00 p.m., Nil walked into the room and announced that the doctors had called him on the cell phone, letting him know the colostomy reversal surgery was a success. Gloria and Njeri hugged each other, cried, prayed, and called Mami and Baba in Kenya to give them the good news.

Lucy had hoped to leave the hospital in time to attend her niece Ethel's high school graduation on June 19, 2010. She knew she could not leave the hospital until her bowels began to function.

"Maybe it's just as well because I know you will have all the good food and I won't be able to eat it," she joked.

Lucy was surprised and happy when Ethel, who had decided to end her graduation party early, showed up at the hospital wearing her cap and gown. Njeri, her daughter Jazmine, and their friends Pam and Fred and their three children, Chepi, David, and Jonathan accompanied her. Lucy was overjoyed taking pictures with Ethel.

"See, Aunt Lucy, you didn't miss anything," Ethel said.

The smile on Lucy's face said it all. Lucy was discharged from the hospital the following day; she had passed gas and had a bowel movement as she had hoped.

When Lucy felt well enough, she was ready to leave the house but soon realized that her body would take a while getting used to functioning as it had before cancer. She had to plan her meals carefully because some irritated her bowels more than others. She handled the constant diarrhea and constipation with a sense of humor; she never complained about any of it.

"My butt is on moto, moto fire, fire today," she would respond with a laugh on the days she was having diarrhea.

"My poop is confused about the direction it should go today. My body is still looking for the colostomy bag," Lucy joked when she was constipated. There were very few days when everything was working as it should. "I have noticed that, depending on what I eat, I can either be stuck in the house all day or I am able to venture out," Lucy told Njeri one day.

"I have to plan my meals based on what I want to do for the day. I noticed that vegetables and milk always give me diarrhea. Bread and meats, on the other hand, make me constipated. I have to find a balance." With that, Lucy strove every day to eat healthy and consciously and made this a lifestyle change. With the diet modification, Lucy had freedom to do whatever she wanted to. She discovered that the military gym offered Zumba dancing several times a week; Lucy got hooked immediately.

By the end of July, which was seven weeks after surgery, Lucy was feeling good enough to make a trip to upstate New York to see her sister Lydiah, who now had two children. Lucy kept busy the entire time, helping Lydiah with housework. Most of the days, Lydiah wondered where the energy was coming from; Lucy would say that after spending days bedridden or unable to do any chores, she wanted to accomplish something each day, no matter what that thing was, big or small. Njeri and Gloria drove to upstate New York to pick Lucy up and bring her back to Virginia.

When Lucy returned to Virginia, she started sending out job applications. Even though she kept busy with her many projects, she wanted to be among adults and longed for social connections. The unemployment rate was very high during 2010, so Lucy, like many other applicants, received a lot of rejection letters. Lucy decided to find volunteer work to keep her busy. The assisted living facility a few miles from the house in Quantico was thrilled to have her as a volunteer. Lucy soon found great joy working with older people who were eager to tell their life stories. Volunteering three times a week gave Lucy the break she needed; the folks were eager to see her and looked forward to her visits.

For the latter half of 2010 and the first half of 2011, life returned to normal for Lucy. She spent most of her days making her jewelry, which Njeri sold, and picked up more creative projects. She enjoyed reading and writing.

On the days she was not volunteering, Lucy went to Zumba. On some weekends, she would travel with Nil to North Carolina to visit his son and daughter. On others, she spent time at Njeri's or went shopping or sightseeing. Lucy was enjoying life. She was nervous every time she had to go for a colonoscopy, CAT scan, or MRI to see if the cancer had returned. Fortunately, the tests showed that the chemo treatment was working because the cancer had not spread.

In July of 2011, Lucy, Njeri, and Gloria drove to New York to visit Lydiah, who had an upcoming birthday. They returned to Virginia in time for Lucy's thirty-sixth birthday; Njeri had planned a party for this occasion. In lieu of gifts, Njeri asked the invitees to give cash to help Lucy offset some of the cost for travel to Kenya in August to visit with Mami, Baba, and other family members. Everyone's generosity surprised Lucy. In August of 2011, two years after Lucy was diagnosed with stage IV colon cancer, she was in Kenya, enjoying family; the doctors had predicted she would not last this long. It did not escape Lucy that she was lucky, and she was extremely grateful.

When Lucy returned to Virginia, she was happy to learn that the application she submitted at the Family Health Center of Woodbridge, a military treatment facility, had been reviewed, and they wanted to interview her. Lucy was offered a position on an "as needed basis" with potential for full-time employment. Lucy was overjoyed to return to work and quickly became friends with most of her colleagues; she bonded immediately with her team leader, Tina, whom she affectionately called Teen Tin.

The joy of being gainfully employed was short-lived. In December of 2011, Dr. Delmas called Lucy to let her know that the MRI done a few days prior showed that the cancer had returned, and he wanted to schedule an appointment with Lucy to discuss her options. After the call, Lucy's spirit was crushed; she was crying as she called Njeri, but she quickly recovered and said, "It could be worse. Dr. Delmas said that I have options, so once again, I have to face my fears bravely."

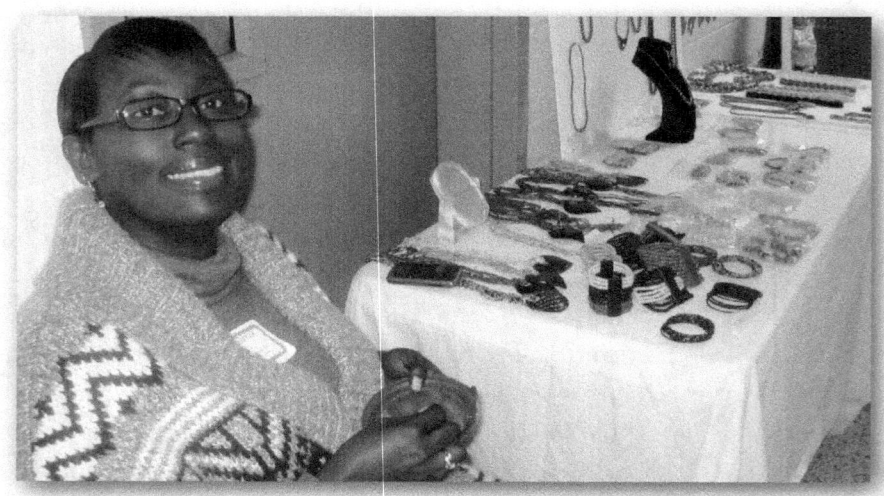

Lucy at a crafts show selling her jewelry

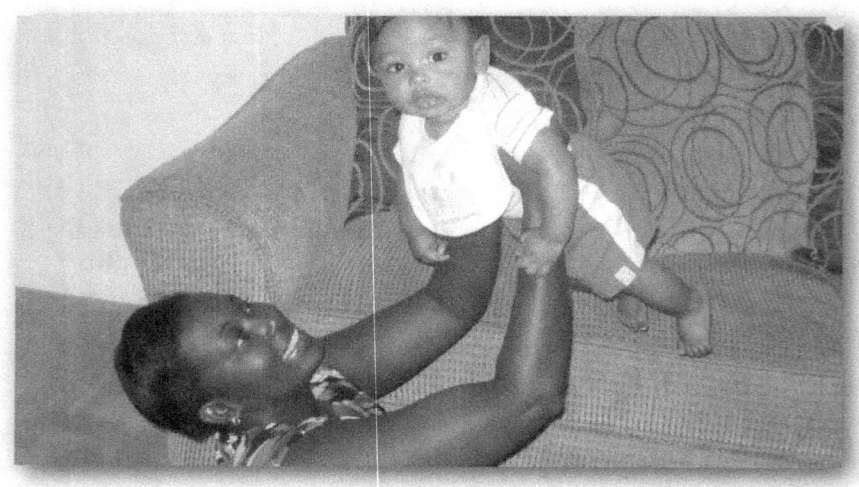

Lucy and Eli

CHAPTER 10

A New Normal

LUCY, NIL, AND NJERI ARRIVED at 8:00 a.m. for the appointment with Dr. Delmas, who had moved from Walter Reed Army Medical Center to the National Naval Medical Center in Bethesda. On this day, Lucy was pensive and seemed in a daze. Dr. Delmas walked in quietly and hugged Lucy and shook hands with Nil and Njeri.

"I am sorry to give you this news, Lucy," Dr. Delmas said.

"I thought I was going to be one of the few that beat this dreadful disease," Lucy responded.

"Chemo worked before, so we will try it again. Because the disease came back, it is very likely that you will be on chemo treatment or some type of maintenance for the rest of your life." Dr. Delmas told Lucy she would start chemo immediately.

Nil did not like the idea of driving to Bethesda twice a week every other week, so he asked if Lucy could transfer to Fort Belvoir Hospital, which was closer to their house. Dr. Delmas offered to talk to oncologists at the Fort Belvoir Army Community Hospital about Lucy's case. Just like before, a schedule was made for Lucy to receive chemo treatment every other Wednesday, take a pump home for slow infusion, and return on Friday to have it removed.

At first, Lucy was apprehensive about leaving the care of Dr. Delmas, whom she had grown very fond of. After a couple of treatments and the back and forth to Bethesda, Lucy decided to transfer to Fort Belvoir under the care of Dr. Verma. After a few visits, Lucy and Dr. Verma formed a superb doctor-patient relationship based on trust, respect, honesty, and a sense of humor.

Lucy considered herself the luckiest cancer patient to have Dr. Verma as her doctor. She announced to everyone who cared to ask how she was that she had the best oncologist in the world.

Getting treatments at Fort Belvoir allowed Lucy to work more hours; her biweekly schedule started with work on Monday and Tuesday, chemo treatment all day Wednesday. Then she took the pump home for slow infusion and returned to work all day Thursday and half a day on Friday. She returned the pump to the hospital on Friday afternoon. The Saturday, Sunday, and Monday following chemo were exhausting, and Lucy could barely walk from the fatigue. During the weekends, Lucy's sisters Njeri, Gloria, Lydiah, and their families would visit Lucy and Nil's house to make sure Lucy was OK. Lucy would quickly bounce back to her energetic self and return to work on Tuesday or Wednesday, a full week after chemo. She would clean, cook, and try to fit everything she needed to on Thursdays, Fridays, and the weekend before starting all over again.

Nil started going out of town on most weekends. At first, Njeri thought he was leaving the house on those weekends to avoid being around Lucy's family. However, one weekend while suffering from chemo fatigue, Lucy told Njeri and Gloria that she had something to show them.

"You will not believe the nerve of this man," Lucy said.

"What is it, sis? You can just tell us what it is without having to get up," Njeri responded.

"You have to see this to believe it. Give me a cup of chai for a boost of energy, and I will show you."

Gloria poured a cup of tea for Lucy, who sipped it slowly. When she was done, Lucy climbed the stairs at a snail's pace and brought back a small white plastic bag. She had a grin on her face.

"On Thursday, I unpacked Nil's bag and found this in it," Lucy said, pulling large blue lace underwear from the bag. "When he came home from work, I asked him who it belonged to; he said he didn't know, and it's likely mine. Of all the stupid shit I've ever heard, this one takes the cake. Can you believe that? He also forgot to log off his e-mail; I found several communications with a woman called Pandora. All this time he travels to North Carolina, pretending my family is chasing him out of the house, he has been having an affair.

"Look at this picture I forwarded to my cell phone. This is Pandora; she sent him an e-mail of herself wearing a bikini. The woman is at least three hundred fifty pounds, and I am almost certain that this is her underwear. I had both her first and last names and a picture so, naturally, I Googled her name and found her on Facebook. I was angry and tempted to post that picture, but I noticed that she was a mother, and I did not have the guts to embarrass her because I believe it's wrong. She may not have known that he is married. I sent her an e-mail to let her know who I was." By this time, Lucy had stopped grinning.

Njeri and Gloria looked at Lucy with concern. Not only was she dealing with chemo, she had a cheating husband. "What will you do, sis?" Gloria asked.

"I told him he can do whatever he wants," Lucy replied. "I'd rather you did not concern Mami and Baba with this foolishness. I don't want to worry them. I can't remember if I read it or if someone told me that some of the spouses with seriously ill partners have affairs as a coping mechanism. I am hoping this is a one-time thing," Lucy continued. "I am not making an excuse for him, but I really don't have the energy to deal with this now. I am going to assume that he is having an affair and live my life one day at a time." Lucy had no desire to discuss the affair further.

Njeri and Gloria accompanied Lucy to Fort Belvoir on the days she had chemo. A few times, when they were unavailable, Nil would take Lucy for chemo, but he might as well have been absent because he would bury himself in his laptop, not saying a word to Lucy or the caregivers. Lucy disliked having Nil in the room while she was getting chemo.

"He has nothing but negative energy," she would complain. After a while, Nil stopped coming to Lucy's treatment altogether. He dropped her off in the morning; Njeri would join her a few hours later, then take her home after chemo.

Six months after Lucy's underwear discovery, Nil was still making his trips out of town on weekends after Lucy's chemo treatments. In July of 2012, Lucy said she needed a break from chemo, so after the scan revealed the cancer cells were shrinking, she asked Dr. Verma if she could take a break. The doctor agreed to have Lucy skip two treatments. Coincidentally, her friend

Tina from work and two other girls were going to Jamaica on vacation. Lucy took advantage of the opportunity to have fun with friends. For a week, Lucy enjoyed the all-inclusive resort, taking advantage of sightseeing, music and dancing, food, and everything else Jamaica had to offer. When she returned to Virginia, Lucy felt invigorated and renewed and ready to face life with whatever challenges it had.

The sense of rejuvenation was short-lived. Nil started accusing Lucy of having an affair while in Jamaica. Lucy confided in Njeri that Nil had started referring to her as a bitch.

"I don't have to take his insults. I have a job, and I can afford to rent my own place. The only problem is that, as a part-time employee, I do not have health insurance. He asked me why I am not yet dead. I think he was hoping that I would die in two years so he could get the life insurance he took out on me. On the days I can't get out of bed due to chemo fatigue, he yells when I don't have dinner ready. He complains when I don't wash clothes. He is already taking money from me to cover house bills every two weeks, even though I make a fraction of the salary he makes," Lucy told Njeri.

What she was hearing appalled Njeri. She asked Lucy to move in with her immediately, and Lucy politely refused, saying she needed to consult a lawyer to see what her options were. Njeri had an acquaintance who had recently divorced her military husband, so she asked for and received the lawyer's contact information. Njeri wrote the lawyer, explaining that her sister Lucy had been married for four years to an active-duty person who would soon retire from the military. Njeri explained that Lucy was looking for legal advice based on the fact that she was undergoing treatment for stage IV colon cancer and only had TriCare military health insurance under her husband who was becoming increasingly verbally abusive and also committing adultery. In the e-mail to the lawyer, Njeri noted that she was concerned that the stress Lucy had to deal with may have been compromising her treatment outcome. The lawyer's office responded immediately, giving Lucy an appointment one day in August 2012 at 11:00 a.m. The consultation fee was five hundred dollars, and Njeri offered to pay.

Njeri drove Lucy to Fairfax, Virginia, to meet with the divorce lawyer; they arrived in the office at 10:45 a.m.; the friendly receptionist gave Lucy paperwork to complete. The lawyer promptly walked in the office at 11:00 a.m. and greeted them. He asked Lucy to come up to his office alone. Njeri sat and waited for an hour before she saw Lucy emerge with red, puffy eyes and a runny nose. Njeri ran toward her sister and gave her a hug. She took the soggy tissues from Lucy's hands and gave her some clean ones from the reception table. Lucy assured Njeri that she was fine and wanted to talk in the car.

"I have to pay the consultation fee," Njeri said.

"He said it's on the house. He will not charge me," Lucy responded. They got into the hot car; Njeri turned the ignition and put the air conditioner on. Lucy composed herself, looked at Njeri, smiled, and started talking.

"When I walked in his office, I told him how I was diagnosed with cancer a year after marrying Nil. I told him that Nil was supportive but always felt that my family was always around. I explained to him that in Kenya, families come first, and he said it is the same with the American culture and most of the world. I told him about the affair I was aware Nil was having and showed him the picture sent to him by Pandora. I told him I was sick and tired of the abuse and I wanted out, but was afraid that I would have no medical insurance. I told him that I love Dr. Verma and his team at Fort Belvoir. If I was to get other insurance, I would not be able to see the same doctors. I also told him that Nil is abusive and is always threatening to file for divorce but never goes through with it.

"The lawyer listened without interrupting, then said it is unfortunate and sad that a man like Nil is just being an asshole. He said legally, if Nil divorces me, then he will be forced to support me, which would help me pay for insurance. However, if I left him, I will have abandoned Nil, and he will owe me nothing. The lawyer said he will file for divorce if that's what I wanted to do, but the adultery claim will not stand in the court of law. He said that unless I catch Nil in bed red-handed, a picture meant nothing. He asked if I knew how much the treatment would cost with private or no insurance, and I told him it would be approximately ten thousand dollars per treatment.

"The lawyer said that I needed to think clearly to figure out if I had the strength to fight Nil and cancer at the same time. He said he would support me and would lower the attorney fees if I chose to go through with the divorce. He asked me if I love Nil, and I told him I did. He told me that if I chose not to file for divorce, it will be agonizing for Nil because he will not be getting his way.

"I am crying because I have decided that I care more about the treatment than I care about him. He can divorce me if he wants, but I am not filing for divorce. Every time he curses at me, I will be thinking 'ten thousand dollars.' I know this sound like I am selling my soul for insurance, but this is my life; I cannot go through the stress of filing for a divorce. I don't sleep with him anyway; I don't care if he brings a woman to his room. He wants his family and his friends to think that the marriage is perfect and that he is a supportive husband. I will play along because I like some of his family members, but in my opinion, he is an evil person and he can do whatever he wants. I have to put all my strength on fighting cancer."

Before leaving the lawyer's parking lot, Lucy called Mami and told her that she would not file for divorce while undergoing chemo. Njeri drove to the nearest shopping mall to get lunch. They enjoyed soup, salad, and the garlic bread at the Olive Garden that Lucy loved.

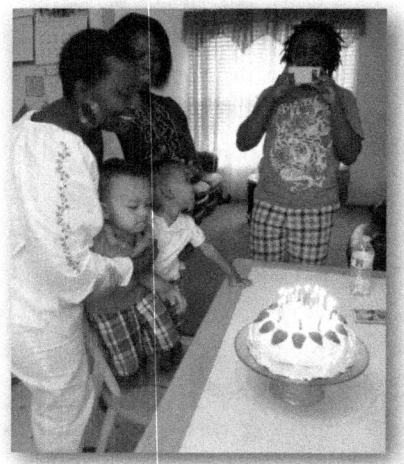

Lucy getting help blowing 37 candles on her birthday

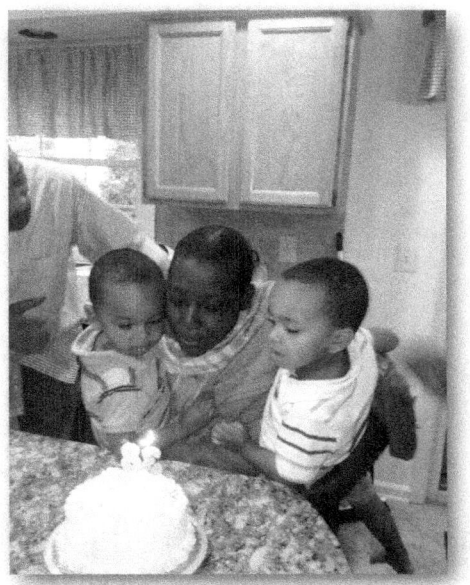

Lucy blowing candles for her 38th birthday with Ethan and Eli

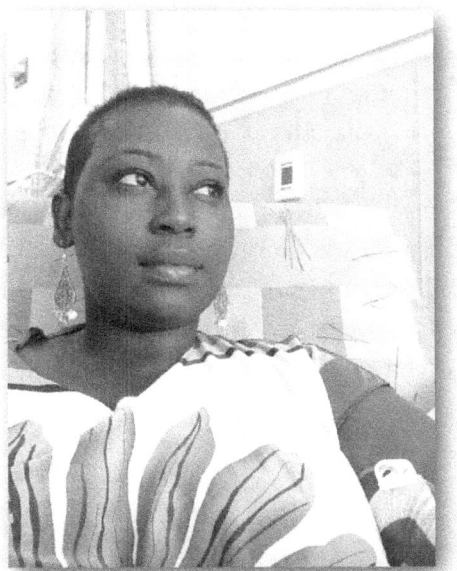

Back on chemo treatment day

CHAPTER 11

One Day at a Time

LUCY WORKED HARD TO FIND peace after the lawyer's visit. She increased her reading from one to two or three books on most days. She read her Bible every morning, marking and memorizing verses, until it was well worn. Aside from the Bible, Lucy read inspiring books and biographies. She made a conscious decision to focus on all things positive and avoided negativity of all kinds, including people she referred to as "energy zappers and joy stealers."

Lucy watched only positive TV programming. She loved Ellen DeGeneres and Oprah Winfrey and tried to get tickets to the shows so she could meet them. She found inspiration in *Good Morning America*'s Robin Roberts, who survived cancer and its side effects, giving Lucy hope that she, too, could recover.

She refused to engage Nil in the arguments he tried to provoke, which made him even angrier. He constantly insulted her, even when she could barely get out of bed, calling her lazy, bitch, black ass, and whatever else he could think of. When he was not insulting her, he would go for days without saying a word to her. Lucy referred to the quiet time and his out-of-town adulterous trips as "freeeeedom time," with an emphasis of the word *free*. She truly felt at peace when Nil was away from her. Lucy understood that each new day was a gift, and she made them count. She literally took it a day at a time.

Njeri, Gloria, Lydiah, and the rest of the family were ever more concerned about Lucy, but she insisted that she was fine. Lucy assured them that, although the verbal abuse hurt, it was only for a moment and she had developed a thick skin. Lucy did not hold any of it back; she would tell her sisters, her friends, and Mami every time Nil went on ugly rants. Njeri noted that this abuse was occurring at least twice a month, and it coincided with the weekends Lucy was recovering from chemo side effects, the moment she was weakest.

One Sunday morning, when Njeri was getting ready to visit Lucy, who was very weak after receiving chemo on the Wednesday before, Mami called Njeri and said she wanted to speak with both her and her husband, Tony. "I just talked to Lucy, and she had not eaten breakfast. She said she was waiting for you," Mami told Njeri.

"I am heading over to her house, Mami. She asked me for *ucuru,* Kenya porridge, which I just finished making," Njeri responded.

"I need to tell you and baba Ethel something I am sure you already know. I have told you before that you are the oldest daughter, you are a good daughter, and I thank God that he gave you to me. I know you have enough responsibilities, but I want to add more because I know you can do all things when God is on your side. You are my daughter, so I also know that you are a strong woman," Mami continued. "I am not there to take care of your sister. If it were up to me, she would be here with me. That will not happen because I know she is getting the best care there. Your sister decided to fight for her life; she didn't want to go on with divorce proceedings because she believes that the psychological and emotional exhaustion, added to the physical exhaustion from chemo, would destroy her. I do not judge her for making this decision, and nobody should. I need you to promise me that no matter how angry you get at Nil, no matter what he says or does to isolate you from your sister, you will not abandon her. You are now the mother, and Tony is the father. I am giving you that responsibility." Mami's voice was breaking with emotions.

"Mami, I will never, ever abandon Lucy or any of my sisters. I promise," Njeri responded.

"I know, but I wanted to hear it from you. I know it's hard for you, Lydiah, and Gloria to see your sister endure verbal abuse, let alone in her condition. I know you have tried to offer her solutions, but it's not in your place. All you sisters can do is continue supporting her. If she ever wants to leave him, support that as well. Let me talk to baba Ethel. I love you," Mami concluded as she always did. Njeri handed the phone to Tony.

"How are you, Baba?" Mami asked Tony. "I want to come there to see my children and you, Baba. I miss you very much." Even with Mami's broken English, the two had developed a language of their own from the time they met when Tony served in Kenya. "Baba Ethel, you are a good man. Lucy is your sister, but I want you to be her father, too," Mami said.

"Mami, I have told Lucy to move in with us, but she wants her independence. I support her. I promise I will look after her and will be there for her," Tony reassured Mami.

Mami called Lydiah and her husband, Mike, and then she called Gloria. Mami wanted assurance that her family was still loyal to one another, even though she knew she had nothing to worry about.

Njeri and Gloria and their children, Ian and Jazmine, went to see Lucy who had left the door opened for them. The sisters walked into the house, fixed a plate for Lucy, and took it upstairs to her. As always, Lucy refused to eat in bed, insisting she was not that sick. She dragged herself downstairs, ate a few spoonfuls of porridge, and fell asleep sitting on the couch. Njeri went upstairs to the linen closet and grabbed a towel and the foot spa she had given Lucy when she could no longer go to a salon for a pedicure. Njeri laid a big trash bag on the floor near the couch where Lucy was sitting. Gloria poured warm water into the small blue foot spa, added bath bubbles and a little Epson salt, and placed the spa near Lucy's feet. Njeri gently took Lucy's foot, folded her pajama pants, and massaged the foot gently. Lucy opened her eyes, smiled, then fell back asleep. Njeri gently washed and dried Lucy's feet one at a time. Gloria had baby oil ready to start massaging. For a while, the sisters massaged Lucy's feet while they continued talking and laughing; Lucy would open her eyes from time to time, responding in agreement or joining in the laughter. As they were finishing, Nil opened the door and walked into the living room.

"You all spoil Lucy," he said and went upstairs to what Lucy called his man cave.

The sisters waited a few hours, and then Gloria prepared a small plate of rice, chicken stew, and cabbage she had cooked at her house. Once again,

Lucy ate a couple of spoonfuls and went back to sleep. As dusk fell, Lucy said she was ready to go back upstairs to sleep. Njeri warmed up a small plate of porridge and asked Lucy to eat slowly. Once again, Lucy ate a few spoonfuls and said she was done. Njeri asked her to try eating the rice and chicken prepared by Gloria. This time, Lucy ate a little more.

She asked Gloria to make Kenya chai. She drank half a cup, stood up, stretched, and with a big grin on her face, said, "*Haya, nindanogoka, nindaigwa wega; ruciu ngathie guteng'era nja,*" which directly translates, "*OK, I am rested. I feel better; tomorrow I will go running outside.*"

As the sisters were leaving the house, Nil walked into the kitchen and mumbled, "There is nothing to eat in this house." Njeri offered him the food that Gloria made. Nil ignored her. The sisters left as soon as Lucy went upstairs to bed.

On Tuesday, Lucy woke up at 4:30 a.m., feeling invigorated. She went through her morning routine of reading the Bible, praying, and listening to her inspirational music. She readied for work, had breakfast, and was in the office by 7:00 a.m.

Lucy loved going to work and waited for the biweekly meetings where employees were asked to bring something to share. The day before the meetings, Lucy had cooked and baked for her colleagues as though she were having a party. Her family and friends were complimentary of Lucy's excellent baked goods, and soon, she was the family baker, a title she relished. Lucy found healthy options to substitute for the foods she liked. Each time she had a breakthrough with a recipe she liked, it became an opportunity to have a tasting with her sisters to get feedback. These constant gatherings turned into actual parties at Njeri's house where they would cook, talk, and dance long after dark whenever Lucy could. By all accounts, Lucy was living her life fully.

One cold night in January of 2013, while they were having one of the gatherings, Njeri received a call from Baba saying that Mami was unwell but did not want to trouble the children because she didn't think it was something serious. Baba was concerned because Mami had not been eating and had lost a lot of weight. The local clinic had diagnosed her with typhoid fever saying the headache, lethargy, diarrhea, and aches and pain she had, were indicative of the disease. After weeks of clinic visits, Baba said Mami was not getting better, and recently, she had been vomiting after every meal. Njeri asked Baba if she could speak to Mami; he said that she was sleeping. He promised to call her the following day when Mami was up.

The call came in when Njeri was at work on a Monday. Baba had accompanied Mami to the clinic, and when the doctor told her she needed rest to give the medicine time to work, Baba had insisted the doctor talk to Njeri. Njeri asked him for his specialty, and he replied he was a health worker, not a medical doctor. Njeri spoke to the health worker for a while, asking about tests and medication Mami had received. Soon, it became clear that Mami was receiving very poor health care.

Njeri called her childhood friend in Kenya, Dr. Githaiga, who had a great love and respect for Mami; he called her immediately and asked that Mami come to Nairobi the following day to see him. Mami agreed to have her son, Jeff, take her to see the doctor in Nairobi. Dr. Githaiga made arrangements for Mami to have several tests that included blood work and a colonoscopy. The results were astonishing; Mami had a large tumor on the walls of her colon. Dr. Githaiga, a respected surgeon, scheduled surgery within days. After surgery and biopsy, the diagnosis was stage II to III colon cancer; she was scheduled to start chemotherapy treatment as soon as she recovered from surgery. The family was numb with shock. Lucy was the one reminding each of her family members that they had something to be grateful for. "Mami is strong," she said. "If anyone can beat this, it will be her." Somehow, the family believed her.

The cost of surgery and chemotherapy treatment for Mami was astronomical by any standards, but even more so in Kenya. The sisters put together funds that paid most of the initial bill; fortunately, another family friend, Anne, was able to arrange treatments for Mami at a radiology clinic she ran, agreeing to discuss cost later. She told Njeri and the family that they could make payments whenever they could. Anne told Njeri that Mami loved and treated her like her own daughter; to her, making treatments available was the least she could do. On a day that could have been depressing, Njeri felt gratitude; all along, Lucy was right it truly could have been worse.

Both Lucy and Mami were undergoing the same chemo regiment every other week. However, while Mami was losing weight, Lucy was gaining weight due to the steroids. Since her twenties, Lucy had not been thin, but rather had toned muscles and a curvy figure. She wondered why all of a sudden she was gaining weight on a weekly basis and going up several dress sizes in a short period of time. Her hair was falling out again, and because she was working, she decided to buy wigs to wear to work. She developed a "moon face," something that made her self-conscious. Her skin pigmentation became almost blue black. At first, she thought that her thyroid levels were low, even though she had been taking Synthroid and was monitored often. Lucy decided to talk to Dr. Verma about her weight gain, but Lucy, as always, found humor in almost everything.

"Dr. Verma, we need to do something about my weight. This morning I couldn't find pants that fit. This is why I am wearing sweatpants," Lucy said to the doctor one Wednesday while getting chemo treatment.

"Lucy, we spoke about this," Dr. Verma responded. "The steroids have this side effect, but you need them. With chemo treatment, unfortunately the moon face and the weight gain go hand-in-hand with some patients."

Lucy stood up and grabbed the upper part of her thigh, "Look, Doc, and be honest with me. Is this thigh not the size of an infant?" Lucy laughed out loudly. Dr. Verma and Njeri couldn't help but laugh with her.

Lucy stopped wearing wigs to work and told her colleagues she would wear scarves and wraps instead. Linda from California, the friend who introduced Lucy to glass jewelry making, whom she affectionately called "my Linda," constantly sent Lucy care packages. Lucy felt a kinship to Linda, who was a cancer survivor. In one of the care packages, Lucy found multiple scarves that matched every outfit she had. One rainy March Monday morning, two days before the next round of chemo, Lucy arrived at work feeling great. She wore a black and white scarf, a polka dot black and white sleeveless dress, a light sweater, and four-inch high-heeled black boots. On this day, her work colleagues all decided to wear scarves, women and men. Lucy was touched and cried openly, not caring who saw the tears.

As with many cancer treatment patients, Lucy's skin started drying and cracking. The cream that Dr. Verma prescribed relieved the discomfort for a while. Lucy's itching bald head became intolerable; she would go in the back at work, remove the scarf, scratch her scalp, apply cream, and put the scarf back on. A few weeks after this routine, Lucy was tired of covering her head. One off-chemo Saturday morning in late April, Lucy marched into Njeri's house dressed as though she had an important event to go to. Her makeup was applied lightly, her lips were shiny from the lip gloss, she sported long silver earrings, and her eyes were bright and beautiful.

"Today is a great day. I am ready to enjoy it. Let's roll," Lucy announced as she walked in.

Njeri stared at her sister, wondering how she did it. *A week ago*, she thought, *Lucy was lying in bed, unable to move. Today, her skin is glowing, her smile is infectious, and she is full of energy.* On this day, cancer was not an issue at all.

Njeri hugged Lucy and said, "Sit down, sis, and don't move. I'll be right back." Njeri ran to the bedroom to grab her phone. "I want this moment, so when you are not well, I can remind you how you felt on a day like this." Njeri snapped a few pictures before they left to go to the mall for shopping. Lucy stopped covering her head that day. Her new favorite song was India Arie's "I am Not My Hair."

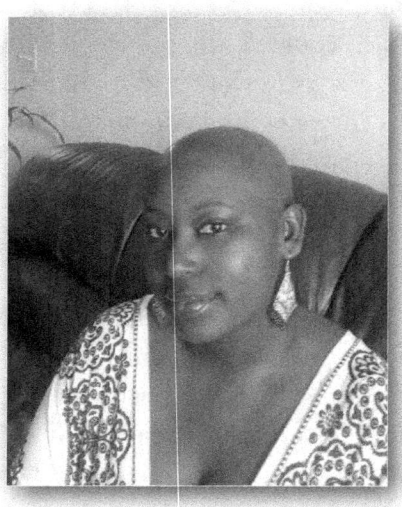

No more wigs or scarves

CHAPTER 12

Take the Good with the Bad

FOR MOST OF 2013, LUCY focused on getting her business products and ideas into fruition. She also decided to make the best out of the dysfunctional marriage she and Nil had. On some occasions, Nil would be supportive of Lucy's ideas and even encourage her to pursue them; other times, he told her bluntly that she was wasting her time and money. Lucy was convinced that Nil was suffering from some form of mental disorder; she encouraged him to seek medical attention, but he refused. Lucy became resigned to Nil's mood swings, as she had no control over them, so there was no need to try to change him. Lucy learned to go with the flow; she was too tired to fight, so when Nil was in a good mood and wanted to indulge her, Lucy obliged.

Njeri, Gloria, Lydiah, and their families stayed away whenever Lucy told them that Nil was behaving; they didn't want to ruin the moment. Some of Nil's actions complicated the relationship between Nil and the sisters. On some weekends when he was not out of town, Nil would barbecue and cook an excessive amount of food, then have Lucy invite the sisters over to eat.

"Are you sure the food is not poisoned?" Njeri asked jokingly one day.

"Who knows?" Lucy responded.

There were times when Lucy was not able to keep the work routine due to pain and exhaustion. Dr. Verma monitored her closely during these periods and, on occasion, would order her to take time off from work. Fortunately for Lucy, her employers at Dumfries Health Center were quite accommodating.

Some of Lucy's colleagues, led by her faithful friend Tina, visited her at home when she went for long periods without working. Lucy always had a positive attitude; she refused to let her work colleagues feel sorry for her, so she never talked about her marriage to them except very rarely to Tina.

Nil retired from the military and wanted to move to North Carolina; Lucy refused. The idea of leaving her doctors and family scared her. By this time, Nil was having a full-blown affair with another woman in North Carolina, Yanna Merde, whom he met before he married Lucy. Lucy believed that Nil wanted to move to North Carolina to be close to Yanna; Lucy thought this was the break Nil had been looking for. Lucy firmly refused to move to North Carolina; for her, this would be the last straw. Lucy did not have a plan B; however, she would not allow herself to be separated from those who cared for her the most. Lucy didn't know what made Nil change his mind, except that a private government contractor in Northern Virginia offered him a position and he had decided to try it for at least a year.

One morning, while Lucy was getting ready to go to work, Nil's mobile phone, which he had left on the kitchen counter, continuously rang. Lucy noticed the 704 North Carolina telephone area code and picked the phone up, thinking it was an emergency from Nil's family. The woman at the end of the line said hello, then hung up when Lucy responded. Lucy saved the number on her cell phone, blocked her caller ID, and called the woman back.

"Hello, I am calling on behalf of Nil. He can't come to the phone right now. May I take a message for him? Who is this?" Lucy said.

"My name is Yanna. I am trying to reach him. I have an important message."

"I know your name. I have seen your e-mails; do you know he is married?" Lucy asked.

"I know he is married, but he told me you have terminal cancer and you will soon die. If I were you, I would spend time with him instead of family. He hates that your family is always at the house. He can't stand it," Yanna responded.

"Be careful what you wish for. You don't know what you would do if you had cancer. Good-bye." Lucy hung up the phone. She was upset because she had just confirmed that Nil was waiting out what he saw as her imminent death. She knew that Nil would be coming downstairs soon, so she went to her bedroom, called Njeri, and relayed the story.

"I can't believe that a grown woman with children would be so cruel. She didn't mince words; she is part of the plan. They are waiting for me to die, sis," Lucy cried. "He is waiting on the insurance money he took out on me."

"Maybe you should reconsider the divorce, sis," Njeri responded.

"No, I will piss them off by staying alive." Lucy was giggling. "Oh well, it's not like I didn't suspect this. Let him plan as much as he wants to. I know that if he collects that insurance money, he will still be an unhappy little man. This woman thinks she has something to look forward to. She will be as miserable as he is. Anyway, I have to go to work. I love you, sis. See you later. Don't worry. I am fine. I have a bigger fight than to worry about a sorry-ass woman who thinks she has found the rich man of her dreams. I have no doubt that she will find out one day."

Before Nil started his new job, Lucy accompanied him for a day of shopping for civilian work clothes. Lucy admittedly loved these moments of married-couple normalcy, even though she understood they were illusions; somehow, they made her imagine what their marriage could be.

October 27, 2013, was the weekend before her fiftieth round of chemotherapy treatment; Lucy joined her sisters Gloria, Njeri, and Lydiah for AIDS Walk DC, a charity event that was dear to them all. This was the second time that Lucy was able to attend this event. Even though the 5k walk made her exhausted at the finish line, Lucy danced alongside everyone else to the drag performances of Beyonce, Tina Turner, Diana Ross, Prince, and others. After the event, Lucy was inspired to dress as Diana Ross for Halloween. She reached out to her old friend Shandra, and together, they came up with an outfit that Lucy would wear to her job.

On October 30, 2013, Lucy spent the entire day getting infused to fight the disease. She noted on her Facebook page, "*So, I realized that today marks round fifty of chemotherapy since I started this journey four years ago. I am blessed, and God has been so good to me. I love life, and I love all those that have been on my side and supported me. I refuse to let cancer CONTROL MY LIFE. I'm not giving up; I know I have a long life ahead of me!"*

The following day, Lucy dressed and felt like Diana Ross; on that day, nothing could bring Lucy down, not even cancer.

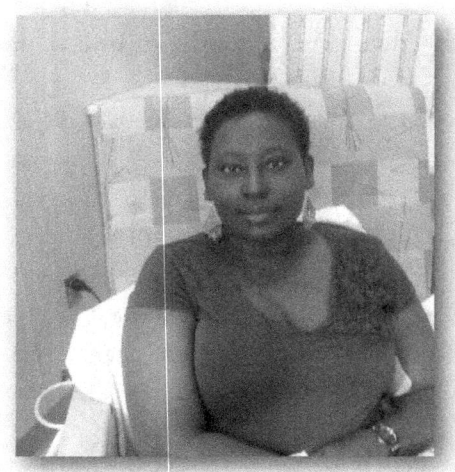

Lucy waiting for another chemo treatment to begin

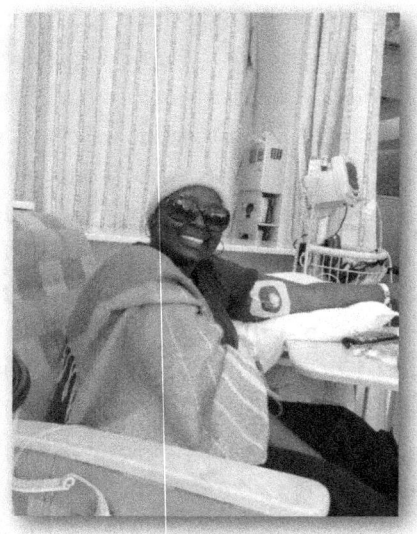

Lucy Joking while getting chemo

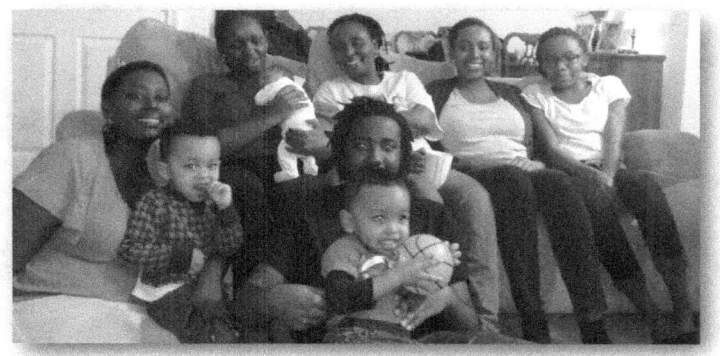

Visiting Lydiah after Zeke's birth

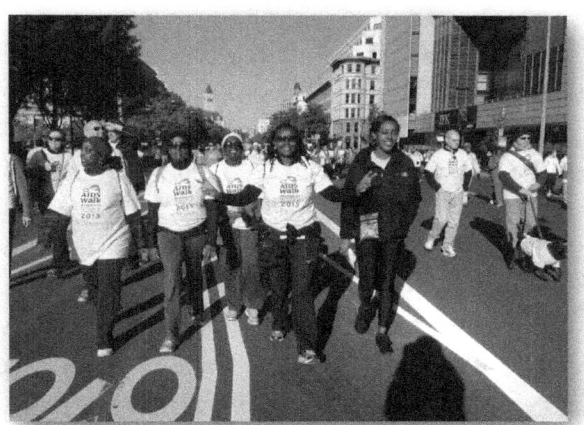

Aids walk 2013 with Gloria, Njeri, Lydiah and Ethel

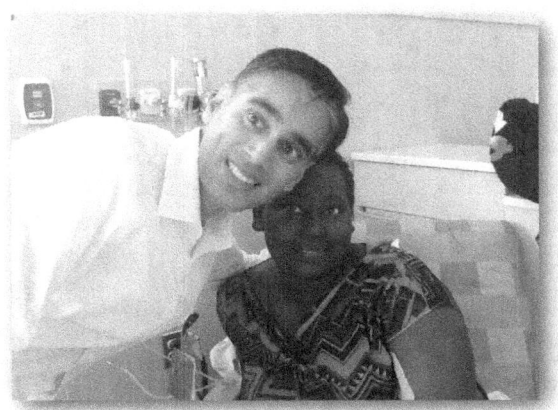

Lucy with her beloved Dr. Verma

CHAPTER 13

I Can Do All Things

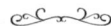

BY THE END OF 2013, Lucy was experiencing frequent abdominal pain. She tolerated the pain as much as she could but occasionally took the painkillers that Dr. Verma prescribed. She hated that the pills made her constipated, and when she tried to correct the problem, she would end up with diarrhea. Lucy also started experiencing occasional dizziness and severe nosebleeds.

For the Thanksgiving holiday in 2013, Lucy once again was the family baker; she baked enough sweets to feed a village. The weekend before Christmas, Njeri and Ian, their nephew, stopped by to check on Lucy since it was the Saturday after chemo and Nil was on his rendezvous in North Carolina once again. Lucy took a while getting downstairs to open the door. She went straight to the couch and fell asleep before Njeri could warm up some food. While Njeri and Ian were waiting for her to wake up, they decided to put up Lucy's Christmas tree, something she always did but had skipped this year. Lucy woke up, saw the tree, and her face lit up.

"I didn't have the energy to put up the tree this time," she said. "When I asked Nil to help bring in my decorations, he said it was too much work and a waste of time."

"Enjoy the tree, Aunt Lucy," Ian said. "I will come by to take it down after Christmas."

Lucy took a few bites of the food Njeri had warmed up for her. She then told Njeri she wanted to take a shower but didn't want to do it while she was alone at the house. Njeri asked Lucy to come over to her house and stay with her until the effects of the chemo wore off, but Lucy declined the offer.

Njeri went upstairs, drew Lucy a bath, and waited while Lucy took her time bathing.

"I've been thinking, sis. I need to go see Mami," Lucy announced. "She is not able to travel, but I can. I will ask Dr. Verma if I could visit for a couple of weeks and take a short break from chemo. I really need to see her."

"I wish I could come with you, sis, but I can't afford to travel this soon after the last trip," Njeri responded.

"You've been there twice since she was diagnosed with cancer and started treatment," Lucy said. "I don't have money for the airline ticket, but I'll put it on my credit card. Nil thinks I shouldn't do it, but I will."

"That will be expensive, sis," Njeri said.

"I have saved some money from the sale of my T-shirts and jewelry, so I will have spending cash. I am not worried about having a lot of extra cash. After all, I am going home, and I'll have everything I need," Lucy said as she got out of the tub.

December 6, 2013, was a great day, as all days were when Lucy was feeling well. She woke up at 4:30 a.m., read her Bible, said her prayers, and started playing her inspirational song of the day as she did before heading in to the shower. Nil, who slept in a different room, stormed into the main bedroom where Lucy slept and turned off the music. He went into a rumbling tirade, but Lucy ignored him by going into the shower, closing the door, and turning on the water. She returned to the room only to find Nil still fuming for reasons she did not understand. Lucy was silent as she dressed, then went downstairs to fix her meals for the day, which included a fruit smoothie and left over vegetables and chicken. Just as Lucy finished making the smoothie, Nil grabbed the food and dumped it in the sink. Lucy was hurt and speechless; at the same time, Lydiah, who called Lucy every morning before she went to work, could hear Nil's insults. Lydiah asked Lucy to record the conversation.

"You need to clean them dishes before you leave from here," Nil said.

"I am not doing anything," Lucy responded.

"Yes, you are, whatever goddamn shit you got going on."

"Whatever devil is in you today, you need to leave me alone. I haven't spoken to you. I haven't said anything. You find me."

"I can talk to you whenever I want to. Fuck you. You take that devil. I can talk to you. As long as you are in this motherfucker," Nil yelled.

"I tell you what, you will pay for this one day. You will pay for every wrong that you've done to me. You will know that the God I serve, he is a good God. And you will pay for it. All the threatening things you tell me, you will choke me, you will kill me, you will beat me up. You going to pay for all of that," Lucy said.

"As long as your black ass is here," Nil said.

"You call me black because you are so white. You sit there and curse me out. I haven't done anything to you. I haven't said anything to you, but because of my condition, you feel you can threaten me and say you are going to beat me and kill me. We will see that," Lucy continued.

Nil mumbled something as he walked away. Lucy stood up for herself and called him out.

"You go ahead and threaten me the way you threaten me. You do all that. Guess what, everything is recorded, and one day, you will pay for it."

"I don't give a shit," Nil said from a distance.

"You sit there and curse me out like I am nothing. I haven't said anything to you. I don't talk to you. I don't say anything to you."

"As long as you're here, I am going to talk to you," Nil retorted.

"This is my house, too, Nil. This is my house also. The same rights you have, I have them, too."

"As long as you're here, I am going to talk to you. If you don't want me to talk to you, get the fuck out." Nil returned close to Lucy.

"I am not going anywhere. This is my house. As long as my name is Lucy with your last name, I am going to be in this house."

"And I am going to talk as long as I am in this house, too," Nil said.

"Guess what, you have the money as you brag to me. You go ahead and file for divorce. So you will talk to me like I am trash because I cannot afford to file for a divorce. So you will make my life miserable. That's what you want."

"As long as you are in this house, I am going to talk. You have that music blasting at six o'clock in the morning."

"You curse me out at six o'clock in the morning, throw my food in the trash. I haven't done anything."

"Don't you have something to do? Go away." Nil dismissed Lucy.

"I tell you what, one day, you will remember me and you will pay for all this."

"You are dismissed, bye," Nil said as he walked away.

Lucy picked up her bag, got into her car, and left for work. When she arrived at the parking lot, she called Njeri to tell her how her morning had begun. "I may not be here when it happens, but I know that what goes around comes around. Nil will never find happiness; he will never find peace, and he will never feel love. Somehow, I feel sorry for him," Lucy said and went on with her day a moment at a time, grateful that she was away from the madness. When she went home that evening, Nil had left for North Caroline.

Freedom for the weekend, Lucy thought with a smile.

Lucy spent the last day of 2013 in bed. She told her sisters that she was feeling tired and wanted to rest. When New Year's arrived, Lucy made calls to everyone, wishing them a happy New Year. For the first time, she did not declare that the New Year would be the greatest year. Instead, she told her family that she was grateful to be alive and that God had a plan for her.

Dr. Verma was reluctant to have Lucy go for a long period without chemo treatment. However, he was sympathetic because Lucy had not seen Mami and understood that this was something Lucy had to do. After discussing the best option for Lucy, Dr. Verma decided to have her take chemo on the Wednesday as usual but adjusted the dosage to limit exhaustion. Lucy bought a ticket for mid-January of 2014.

"I can do all things, through Christ who strengthens me," Lucy quoted Philippians 4:13 whenever Njeri, Gloria, and Lydiah told her they were worried about her making the trip so soon after chemo. Lucy was going to see Mami in Kenya no matter what. She left on the Thursday, a day after chemo, and was scheduled arrived in Nairobi, Kenya, twenty-three hours later.

The family in Nairobi eagerly waited to welcome Lucy when she arrived. Her sister Nancy, her brother Jeff, nephews Waititu and Koki, and nieces Julie and Nina were waiting at the airport when she arrived shortly before midnight. Also waiting were her brothers-in-law Maish and John who had gone to find her when she considered eloping as a teenager. Lucy was filled with joy when she saw them as she exited the airport. Mami waited at the house in Nairobi, while Baba had stayed at the farm in the country; Lucy would see him in a couple of days. As she would say, the long trip was worth it.

Lucy cried as she hugged Mami, who was all smiles. Lucy was surprised to see how much weight Mami had lost. She couldn't have been more than one hundred pounds. The effects of chemo, which included the darkening of the skin, tongue, and hands, were showing on Mami, even though she had completed the treatment a few months before. Mami told Lucy that her feet stayed numb, and sometimes she couldn't tell whether she had shoes on or off until she looked down at her feet. As they chatted, Mami's eyes teared up, but she never cried. Even at her weakest, Mami had to be strong for her child Lucy. Right before dawn, they fell asleep only to wake up a few hours later. When Lucy woke up, Mami was not in her bed. Lucy made her way to the kitchen to find Mami busy making breakfast. She no longer moved with strength, and her step indicated that she was in pain.

"Mami, what are you doing? There are many people in the house. You shouldn't be straining yourself," Lucy scolded her.

"Lucy, don't worry. I wanted to make your favorite porridge," Mami said.

"But I can see you are in pain. Remember, you barely had any sleep and now you are moving around. You need to give your body time to heal," Lucy said.

"I tried to stop her, Aunt Lucy, but she is just like you, hardheaded. I can make the porridge. *Cucu* taught me how to prepare it," Nina her niece jumped in.

"As long as I am able to move and do some work, I refuse to lie down and waste a day that I am grateful to see," Mami said. "There have been days when all I could do was sleep and have others take care of me. I never want to go through that again."

"I know where I get my attitude from. Like mother, like daughter." Lucy laughed.

Two days later, Lucy and Mami made the trip up country to the farm to see Baba. He had prepared a meal for them and was excited to see Lucy. Baba wanted to show Lucy the house she had helped build. Lucy was disappointed that it hadn't turned out the way she thought. The builder had taken advantage of Mami's illness. Lucy and Baba agreed to halt the builder's work and find someone else. They all had a lot of catching up to do, and once again, it was very late when they finally went to bed.

By all accounts, the trip to Kenya went well during the first two weeks. One morning after breakfast, Lucy felt faint and unsteady after suddenly standing up. She sat back down until the dizzy spell ended. She dismissed the feeling thinking she had stood up too quickly and hadn't slept well. However, the dizzy spells happened several times in the following days. One afternoon, Lucy planned to go for shopping with her niece Nina. As she walked towards the car, she stumbled; the driver caught her before she fell. The family was very concerned and urged Lucy to go to the hospital. She agreed to do so, but first, she called Dr. Verma, who told her to get a scan at a hospital in Nairobi and have them send him the results. Anne, the family friend who had helped care for Mami, made arrangements to have the scan done. The results were inconclusive; the dizzy spells continued. Fortunately, Lucy had only one more week in Kenya, and she would soon be returning to her doctor, who would perform more tests.

Two days after arriving back to the United States, Lucy went to Fort Belvoir to take a blood test and get an MRI before seeing Dr. Verma. The MRI results showed that the cancer cells had spread significantly. Dr. Verma told Lucy and Njeri that she was very sick and that treatment would need to be aggressive. While undergoing the treatment, Lucy tried to keep working but was sick on most days. Recently, she had started getting severe nosebleeds and had a chronic cough. By April, Dr. Verma asked Lucy to stop working and give her body time to rest. Lucy had no choice but to resign from her beloved job at the Dumfries Health Center. The supervisor told her that when she felt better, they would be happy to have her back.

Staying home and doing nothing was not an option. Lucy returned to her love of jewelry making. On her Etsy profile, she wrote:

I was diagnosed with stage IV colon cancer in 2009. I was only thirty-four years old when I was diagnosed. I have worked on and off for the past five years, but it's been absolutely hard, but since I don't like to be idle, I kept working, sometimes even eight hours a day. Finally, my doctor demanded that I quit working for a while because I was straining my body too hard plus I'm still on chemotherapy. I love crafting, and I tried various things, but I always go back to beading. I love the joy I get once I finish and look at the finished product. Making jewelry enables me to forget what's going on inside my body; I can go for hours doing my jewelry. I love the fact that my customers will be proud and will look fabulous once they wear my pieces.

Lucy designed and sold inspirational T-shirts for extra income. Her sisters found new customers who were inspired by Lucy's story. Lucy continued to support the children in Kenya even after she stopped working. She looked forward to spending time with her friends and was pleasantly surprised when her childhood friend Pauline came to visit her in May. When another friend, Tamara, had a birthday, she celebrated by taking Lucy and Pauline to lunch. Lucy was so happy to get out of the house.

By June, Lucy had no appetite and felt as though the food wasn't going down as it should. The persistent cough was becoming a nuisance. After some tests, her doctors decided to drain fluid from her lungs. She felt better after the procedure but still had difficulty eating. A friend suggested that she take medical marijuana to help with her appetite. Dr. Verma told Lucy that he could not prescribe it and that it was illegal. One of the few weekends when Nil was being kind, he asked Lucy to accompany him to North Carolina for a family reunion trip. When Lucy returned, she told Njeri that she had been given some marijuana and had been able to eat.

"People shouldn't be so quick to judge, especially when they have not experienced an illness like cancer," Lucy told Njeri.

In July, Njeri celebrated her fiftieth birthday. Gloria, Lydiah, and Njeri's friends cooked the meal for the fifty invited guests. Lucy made all the appetizers and desserts for the party. The family had a great time with Lucy dancing and learning new steps from friends. Hours into the party, Njeri noticed that Lucy was sitting on the side with a shawl wrapped around her shoulders and was coughing.

"Would you like to go inside, sis?" Njeri asked Lucy.

"No, I am fine. I am a little tired, but nothing hurts: Hey, I should have a party for my thirty-ninth birthday. This is fun," Lucy said, changing the subject.

"It's not too late to plan, sis. We can still have your party. Give me a date that works for you," Njeri said.

As the month progressed, Lucy's stomach pain got worse. She also started having severe back pain. She was taking prescription painkillers more than she wanted to; she worried that some could be addictive. She had difficulty driving but was determined to visit her sister Lydiah in Maryland to celebrate her birthday, which came a week before Lucy's. As expected, Nil was in North Carolina, visiting his woman for the weekend. Njeri drove to Lydiah's; during the visit, Lucy stayed in bed mostly and said that the pain was excruciating. She barely ate the dinner the sisters cooked. The sisters spent the night and stayed until late the following afternoon.

July 29 was Lucy's thirty-ninth birthday. It was also a workday, and Lucy had decided that she would have her party on August 16, in order to give friends and family ample time to attend. Gloria, Njeri, Ethel, Jazmine, and Ian planned to surprise Lucy on her birthday. They knew that Nil would be home but decided to go anyway.

Nil opened the door and asked, "What are you doing here?"

"We won't stay long," Njeri responded. "We wanted to surprise Lucy on her birthday."

"Luuucy, your family is here," Nil yelled and, without saying another word, returned to his office.

Lucy slowly walked downstairs; she hugged her family, then sat down at the kitchen table. She wasn't expecting them to show up but was very happy that they had. Her joy was interrupted by grimacing, frowning, and other distorted facial expressions whenever the pain got worse. She had not taken the pain medicine because it made her sleepy and constipated, she said.

"Have you eaten, sis?" Gloria asked Lucy. "You should eat some vegetables and take the pain medicine."

"I can't eat anything; I tried to drink a protein shake. Don't worry, sis. I'll eat a piece of my birthday cake."

Njeri placed the numbers three and nine on the small vanilla cake they had purchased from the store. Ian lit the candles, and they sang happy birthday.

"Make a wish, Aunt Lucy," Jazmine said.

"Make a wish first or blow the candle first?" Lucy asked.

"Make a wish first," Ethel responded.

Lucy fell silent for a few seconds, then blew the candle. "From my mouth to God's ears," she said, smiling.

The family stayed for twenty minutes, then left to allow Lucy to rest. As they walked out, Nil sneered at them and mumbled some words. The family ignored him and left. Had he known that this would be the last time Gloria, Ian, Ethel, and Jazmine would step into his house, he would have been smiling. Despite all the planning for the big party, these would be the last candles Lucy blew out.

For Lucy, the days following her thirty-ninth birthday were filled with uncertainty. She was able to drive short distances to visit with her sisters as much as possible. One day while visiting, Lucy noticed that Njeri's hair locks needed to be retwisted. Lucy had been twisting Njeri's locks for the past four years and had become an expert in this art. Lucy asked Njeri to come by her house one evening after work so she could do the hair. They agreed that Tuesday, August 12, 2014, would be a good day.

Njeri called Lucy before making her way to the house. Lucy was sleeping and took time to answer the phone. When she did, she sounded very weak, and Njeri was concerned.

"Hey, sis, I don't think I'll be able to twist your hair. I am in so much pain," Lucy said.

"Did you take your medicine?"

"Yes, I did. It's not working anymore," Lucy responded. "I haven't had a bowel movement, and even though I feel like passing gas, nothing is coming out. I know I'll feel better once I use the bathroom."

Njeri was concerned and felt that this time Lucy was seriously ill. Over the years, the sisters had seen Lucy's high tolerance for pain, and they knew that she admitted to feeling it only when it was very intense. Njeri drove over to see Lucy. Nil opened the door and gave Njeri a blank stare; Njeri ignored him. She ran upstairs to find Lucy lying in bed in a fetal position.

"We should go to the emergency room, sis," Njeri suggested.

"It's just that my stomach is bloated. That's where the pain is coming from. Dr. Verma gave me some medicine, and I promised him I will go to the hospital if I feel worse. If it continues, I will go to the emergency room. Maybe if I drink something, I'll be able to go."

"Take some of your chocolate protein shakes. I'll get one from the kitchen," Njeri said as she headed to the door.

"I don't have any left, sis."

Njeri drove to the store and bought a six pack of Ensure protein shakes and returned to Lucy's house. Lucy liked the shakes cold, so she put ice in a glass and headed upstairs. Lucy took a sip of the shake and told Njeri she couldn't take any more. Njeri gently massaged her stomach. Lucy turned her back away from Njeri and passed a sustained and malodorous emission.

"You'd better run, sis," Lucy said, laughing. "This one is like tear gas."

"You are right, sis. This one is making my eyes water." Njeri was laughing so hard she had tears in her eyes.

Lucy had two more emissions; Njeri had to leave the room. Lucy felt better and walked Njeri downstairs to the door. Nil peeked from the office to see what was going on, but they ignored him. This would be the last time Njeri stepped into his house. Three days later, Lucy called Njeri to let her know that she was throwing up and had called Dr. Verma who told her to go to the emergency room. She had called Nil to take her, and he was on his way.

Njeri was at work miles away; she felt helpless, as she had to wait until evening for transportation to take her to her sister. This time, Njeri felt in her gut that it was different. She decided to take a walk, as she felt tears welling up in her eyes. As she crossed the street, she heard a car honking and realized she had not looked before she stepped on the road. From a distance, she heard someone call her name. She looked to see her friend Nicole pushing her bike.

"Where are you going so fast?" Nicole asked. Njeri burst into tears without saying a word.

Nicole led Njeri to a bench in a small park near the street. She listened as Njeri told her that Lucy was going to the hospital and that this time Njeri was really frightened. Nicole calmly spoke to Njeri about sickness, fear, and anxiety. She read a few verses from the Bible and reminded Njeri that no matter what, God was in control and all Njeri could do was to trust Him. At that moment, Njeri knew that Nicole was a divine intervention; she was no longer afraid.

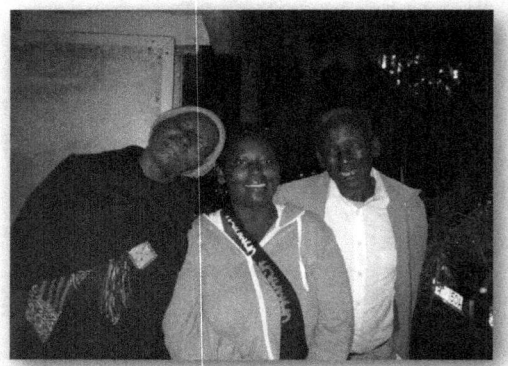

Last picture with Mami and Baba at Jomo Kenyatta airport

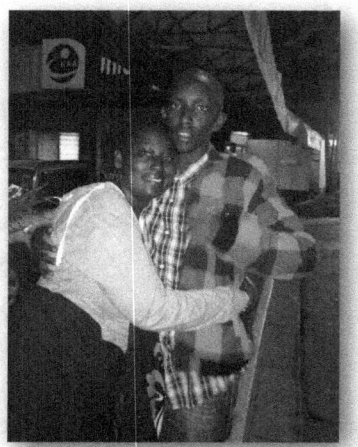

Last Picture with Jeff

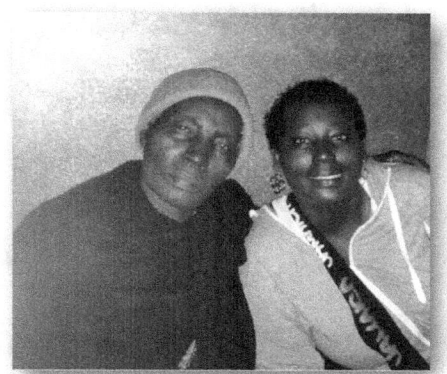

Last Picture with Mami at the airport

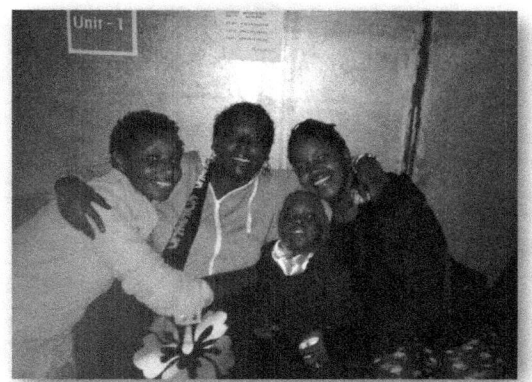

Last picture with Julie, Nisey and Nina

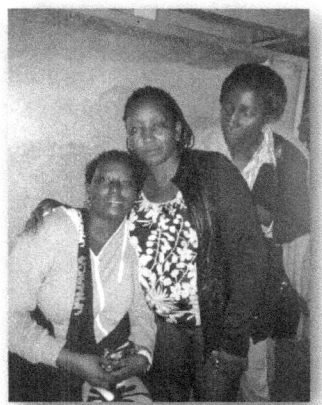

Last picture with Nancy and cousin Susan

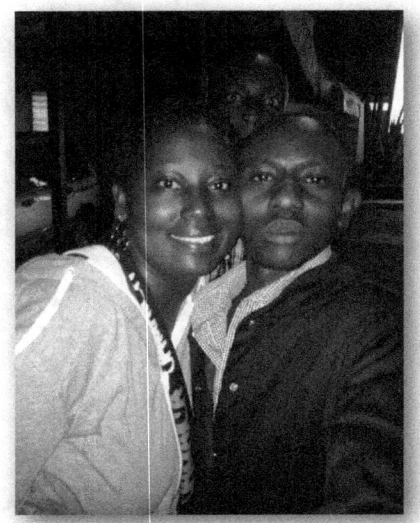

Last picture with nephew Waititu

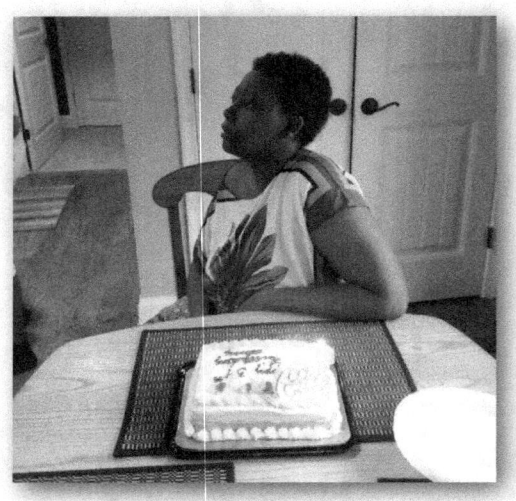

Last birthday cake on July 29, 2014

CHAPTER 14
Hospital Admission

NJERI ARRIVED AT FORT BELVOIR Army Medical Hospital in the evening to find Lucy in bed hooked to a nasogastric tube known as an NG tube. The tube was being used to decompress the intestinal obstruction. Nil was sitting in the room beside her. Lucy told Njeri that the tube was uncomfortable, but it was temporary. Nil told Njeri that the doctors had diagnosed Lucy with bowel obstruction as a result of tumors in her colon and they were considering an operation. As they sat in the room, multiple doctors and nurses walked in and out, talking to Lucy and asking questions.

Lucy's answers were the same. "No, I haven't had a bowel movement since Sunday. The last time I passed gas was three days ago. No, I haven't been able to eat anything for a week. I started throwing up this afternoon."

Two doctors walked in and introduced themselves as surgeons. One of the doctors said he was a gastrointestinal surgeon. The doctors wanted to do a rectal exam to determine if Lucy had a fecal impaction.

"Let me see your hands," Lucy said unexpectedly. Both doctors showed Lucy their hands.

"I want you to do the exam," Lucy said, picking the slimmer hands. "No offence to you, but I don't play that." Lucy was smiling.

Njeri laughed and thought, *This is typical Lucy, finding humor in a very serious situation.*

The doctors decided to admit Lucy. She was transferred to a room on the sixth floor where a stern-looking, no-nonsense nurse, Ms. May, was waiting. Ms. May went through her routine with precision, ensuring that Lucy was comfortable. Nil went home after the admission. Ms. May provided Njeri with a warm blanket and sheets for the pull-out bed in the room. The two barely slept because of the constant checks by nurses. By morning, both Lucy and Njeri had fallen in love with Ms. May for her caring.

Njeri and her girls had planned a trip to New York City that was to last five days starting on the eighteenth of August; back in May, she had asked Lucy to join them to try to meet one of her idols, Robin Roberts of *Good Morning America*, but Lucy had declined, saying it would be too hot for her. Njeri wanted to cancel the trip because Lucy was in the hospital, but Lucy would not hear of it. Her friend Pauline was in town, and Gloria and Lydiah were around, too. Njeri hesitantly left for the New York trip after Lucy convinced her it would make her sad if Njeri cancelled.

Lucy called Njeri several times a day to update her with what the doctors were saying. At some point, they made a decision not to do the operation. Dr. Verma consulted with others to come up with the best solution for Lucy. On Tuesday evening, Lucy called Njeri and told her that Dr. Verma wanted to meet with her and Nil. Lucy did not know what Dr. Verma wanted to discuss, but she said that he insisted that Lucy have someone else with her during this meeting. Lucy and Nil met with the doctors that Wednesday.

Njeri was walking in Time Square when Lucy called. She could barely hear her but knew that Lucy was crying. Njeri asked Lucy to give her a half an hour to get back to the hotel to call her back.

"Hey, sis, what's wrong?" Njeri asked Lucy when she was finally able to call her.

"It's not good news, sis," Lucy replied. "They told me that this is terminal, and I have three months left."

Njeri was quiet for a long time; she knew she had to be strong for Lucy. Lucy broke the silence.

"I am scared, sis. I don't want to die. Dr. Verma said that there is a very slim chance that chemo could shrink some tumors, buying me a little time. I will take that chance."

"Sis, remember that it's not over until God says it's over," Njeri finally said.

"I want to wait until you get back so we can decide how to tell the family."

Njeri returned to Virginia two days later and drove straight to Fort Belvoir. She knocked before entering Lucy's room because she heard voices in the room indicating that doctors or nurses were with her. Lucy's eyes lit up, and she sat up on the bed.

"My sister is here," she said, clapping her hands. The sisters tightly hugged, and then Njeri stepped aside to allow the nurses to finish what they were doing. Lydiah walked in shortly after Njeri's arrival; she was coming to spend the night with Lucy.

"I am so glad to see you guys. Gloria is working tonight, but she's been here every day. I wanted you all to be here together so we can talk."

"OK, sis. I am here for the weekend if you want to wait for Gloria tomorrow," Lydiah said.

Nil walked in as Lucy was explaining to her sisters how uncomfortable the NG tube was. The sisters said hello, to which Nil nodded without saying a word. He stood next to Lucy and said, "Have you told them?"

"Told us what?" Lydiah asked.

"The doctors said she has three months to live," Nil said, looking at Lucy, who started crying. Lydiah reached out, hugged Lucy, and cried.

"Why did you do that, Nil?" Lucy's voice trembled.

"Whether they like it or not, it's happening." Nil seemed to gloat as he spoke.

"Nil, stop. What is wrong with you?" Njeri yelled.

Nil continued to speak. Njeri wrapped her arms around Lydiah and Lucy and started singing one of Mami's songs loudly in Kikuyu. Soon, both Lydiah and Lucy joined her in the song, which drowned Nil's voice. He walked out, muttering words the sisters could not hear. A few minutes later, he came back to the room and asked to see both Njeri and Lydiah outside. Lucy gestured to the sisters to go along, and they did.

"You all need to plan for the worst and stop pretending she will not die," Nil said.

"We know she is very sick, but she is still here. The least you can do is respect her wishes," Njeri said. "Lucy is not stupid; she understands what is going on. We will do what she wants."

"If you don't do it, then I will plan her burial by myself. I asked her what she wanted, and she doesn't seem to know."

"Or maybe you are not listening to her," Lydiah retorted.

"She's my wife, and I have the right to do whatever I think is best for her," Nil said as he walked away from Lydiah and Njeri.

"Run, you punk. That's what you do best," Lydiah said in a combative voice, walking beside him. "This is what you wanted you, small-minded asshole."

"Lydiah, he is not worth it. Leave him alone." Njeri grabbed Lydiah's shoulder so she could stop following. Njeri could see that Lydiah was getting ready to pounce on Nil.

"Yeah, call me a punk, but that doesn't change the fact that she's going to die," Nil said as he walked away from the sisters.

Njeri and Lydiah returned to the room to find Lucy the angriest they had ever seen her. She still wanted to meet the following day as agreed with Gloria in attendance. That evening, Nil did not return to Lucy's room. Lydiah and Lucy talked late into the night, avoiding the topics of Nil and the terminal cancer.

CHAPTER 15

We Will All Die

NJERI AND GLORIA ARRIVED IN Lucy's room that Saturday morning and found Lucy and Lydiah waiting. After the hugs, Lucy started telling Gloria about Nil's behavior the night before. The conversation went on for a while with the sisters feeding off one another. Njeri knew focusing on Nil was a waste of time, so she changed the conversation by establishing a new rule. From here on, Lucy was allowed to vent her anger and frustration about Nil for a few minutes every day, but talking about him all the time gave him too much power, something Lucy was not willing to do. Everyone liked the new rule, especially Lucy. The nurse came in to give Lucy her medicine, and as soon as she left, Lucy started talking.

"I don't want us to talk about this anymore, so please let me finish, especially you, Njeri. You always put a positive spin on everything. I wanted us to meet today because I want you to know what I want in case anything happens to me. I haven't finished writing my will, but now I realize how important it is, and I should have done it a long time ago. I thought if I did, it would hasten death, but the truth is, everyone will die. Each one living today will most likely be dead in the next one hundred years.

"I am not afraid to die, but I am worried about the people I love who I will leave behind. I am worried about Mami. She was never the same after Shiku died. I can't imagine the pain she will suffer if I die before she does. I am worried about Baba, too; it's not fair that they should bury their children.

"I know Nil is waiting for me to die. He has insurance on me and thinks his life will be perfect after I am gone. He will go on with his life with Yanna or whichever pathetic woman he thinks will bring him joy and peace. I am not worried about what will happen to him. It's in God's hands.

"I have decided I will not give Nil the pleasure of speaking on my behalf when I no longer can speak for myself. Njeri, I want you to have that responsibility, because I know you will not pull the plug unless you are certain it's the best option. I know you can find advance-directive forms on the Virginia State website. I want you to bring that form to me.

"As for the will, I have started writing it but did not complete it yet. Njeri, I want you to finish the will for me and bring it on Monday so we can have it signed. I want you to try to work with Nil to make my wishes come true. I know you all don't want to have anything to do with him, but I think if you work together, you may be able to forgive him, therefore freeing yourselves. If Nil refuses to be involved, I want Shandra and James to be the executors of the will. I want you guys to have everything that belongs to me, including the furniture I brought with me after my divorce from JV, my diaries, my jewelry, my Thomas Blackshear collectibles, and everything else that is personal to me. The idea of another woman going through my stuff and enjoying things I have worked hard for drives me nuts. Furthermore, I know they would be more meaningful to you.

"I want to be buried in Kenya, next to Shiku. Nil is trying to convince me to talk to some lawyer and sign some papers, but I won't do it. I know he wants to have full control of my funeral so he can have people feel sorry for him and get the attention he craves. I want Mami, Baba, Jeff, Nancy, Julie, Nina, Koki, Waititu, and all our relatives to have closure and to perform a proper burial. I want to have a church service here in the United States for the people who loved me and cared about me.

"I want Jeff, Nancy, and our nieces and nephews to come to the United States to visit. My goal was to sponsor Nina and Nisey to come live with me. To me, Nina is the daughter I never had. If I don't make it, please continue helping the children. I was hoping to someday start a charity that provides school supplies for the children in Kenya; please keep trying. I was hoping that the cure for colon cancer will be found in my time; if not, please keep talking about it so people can be tested. It's really a curable disease if detected early. I wish that you can find ways to contribute to the research like I have.

"You all know that I have been writing my book; I know I have an interesting story to tell. If I don't make it, please complete my story, which I have on my laptop. I also have kept journals, which I want you to have.

"When I am gone, I want you to forgive Nil. Do not hold anger toward him. He is a very troubled man who has no idea how to find peace. He doesn't trust anyone, and that's a shame. I thought he would view me differently but obviously not. I would like you to reach out to him, but if he does not allow you to, let it go and forgive him. Remember, when you forgive him, you free yourself, so in essence, you will be doing yourselves a favor.

"Njeri, I want you to have the will completed by Monday. I've asked some people here to witness it for me. After that, I do not wish to discuss death anymore. I am still here, and as we say, no one knows the time or day death will come, apart from the good Lord. Please bring the kids so I can tell them what I need to. I am feeling tired, so I'll take a nap. Don't leave. I like hearing your voices as I sleep. I hate the silence; it makes me think I am dead already."

The joke made the sisters smile because Lucy was smiling, too.

"Lydiah is planning to spend another night, and Gloria will be here tomorrow. I'll have your will ready on Monday, sis," Njeri said.

"Good, I'll let Anita and Nuk know that I'll need them to come in as witnesses. I have already asked the legal office downstairs, and they said they can notarize it," Lucy said before she dozed off.

CHAPTER 16

Lucy's Last Will
and Testament

ON SUNDAY MORNING, LYDIAH CALLED Njeri to tell her that Nil had come to the hospital saying he needed to know what time the sisters were visiting Lucy because he was tired of not having time alone with his wife. Nil wanted a schedule so he could plan on when to be there to see Lucy. Lucy thought it was absurd that Nil demanded a schedule. After a conversation with her sisters, Lucy resigned herself to the fact that Nil would not let up until he got the schedule. Lydiah found a blank piece of paper and wrote:

Proposed Schedule for Nil to Review 8/24/2014

- Sunday, 8/24: Gloria will get here at twelve noon. Lydiah leaves at 1:00 p.m.; will not spend the night. Njeri is not spending the night or visiting today.
- Monday, 8/25: Njeri is available to spend the day and night. Njeri is available all day.
- Tuesday, 8/26: Njeri is available to spend the day and night. Njeri is available all day.
- Wednesday, 8/27: Gloria is available to visit and spend the night.
- Thursday, 8/28: Gloria is available to visit and spend the night.
- Friday, 8/29: Lydiah is available to spend the night.

- Saturday, 8/30: Lydiah is available during the day and to spend the night. New schedule to be made on this day.
  Please let us know the night you are not spending the night so that whoever is available can.
  Thank you.

Lydiah taped the schedule on the small white erase board that had the names of the staff on duty. It disgusted Lucy, but she said leaving the schedule on the wall might make Nil realize how ridiculous he was. When Nil came to the room, he looked at the schedule and seemed happy that he did not have to come to the hospital at all, as the sisters had all the days covered.

"I want to speak to my wife alone," Nil said, looking straight at Lydiah.

"What is it, Nil?" Lucy asked.

"Do I need a reason to want to speak to you alone?" Nil said sarcastically.

"It's OK, sis. I'll be outside," Lydiah said as she left the room. Nil left the room about half hour later. Lydiah walked in to find Lucy angry.

"He wants me to sign papers giving him power of attorney, and I will not. He wants me to talk to some lawyers, but I refuse. He is so stupid. While he was trying to convince me to do all this, his phone would not stop ringing. I know it was Yanna calling him," Lucy told Lydiah.

"How do you know it's her?" Lydiah asked.

"Because he left his phone on the bed while he went to pee. All the missed calls are from her. He thinks he is so smart because he changed her name on his contact list. I know that number, and I have it saved on my phone so he can't fool me. I almost feel sorry for Yanna; she can't wait long enough for me to die so she can be with Nil. I know she will get what she deserves, but I really don't care," Lucy said.

That Sunday, Njeri sat down to type Lucy's instructions for her will. She had to get the legal verbiage right, so she used her own will as a format. She called and read each paragraph to Lucy and Gloria to make sure it was what Lucy wanted. When she finished, she e-mailed them the draft; Lucy felt it covered what she needed it to. Njeri agreed to be at Fort Belvoir first thing in the morning.

Njeri arrived at Fort Belvoir to find Lucy awake and ready to sign the documents. Lucy wanted to have everything done in Nil's absence because, as she put it, she would have peace of mind that way. She was concerned that if he found out, he would make everybody's life miserable. Lucy read her will silently and said she was ready to sign. The notary and witnesses arrived shortly after, and Njeri left and went to the waiting room near the nurses' station.

THE LAST WILL AND TESTAMENT OF LUCY WAIRIMU GATHUNGU

I, Lucy Wairimu Gathungu, a resident of the Commonwealth of Virginia, and being of sound mind, do hereby make, publish and declare this to be my last Will and Testament, thereby, revoking and making null and void any and all other Last Will and Testament and/or Codicils to Last Wills and Testaments heretofore made by me. All references herein to this will shall be construed as referring to this Last Will and Testament only.

FAMILY CLAUSE

At the time of executing this Last Will and Testament, I am married to Nil. I have no children. The names of my sisters residing in the United States are below:

Njeri Gathungu
Gloria Gathungu
Lydiah Gathungu

RESIDENCY CLAUSE

Having in mind the possibility that I may be temporarily outside of, or simply be absent from the Commonwealth of Virginia, at the time of my death, I elect and hereby declare that this Will and each and every disposition and provision contained herein shall be construed and regulated by and in accordance with the laws of said Commonwealth of Virginia. It is my desire that this Will be probated in the Commonwealth of Virginia, my place of domicile, and that the principal administration of my estate be made in said Commonwealth of Virginia and that none of the assets of my Estate which may be found in my place of domicile be remitted to any other jurisdiction for administration or distribution.

DEBT CLAUSE

I direct that the executors named pursuant to this Last Will and Testament review (as soon after my death as practical) all of my debts and obligations, as soon as practical. The executors shall pay just debts only after the creditor provides sufficient evidence to support their claim.

PRINCIPAL DISTRIBUTION CLAUSE

I give, devise and bequeath to my spouse and my sisters (my "Principal Heirs"), all my personal belongings after payment of all my just debts, expenses and taxes. Specifically, I bequeath my collection of Thomas Blackshear sculptures, personal clothing and jewelry to my sisters Njeri, Gloria and Lydiah who will make sure that my parents, siblings in Kenya, nieces and nephews receive a gift from me.

EXECUTOR APPOINTMENT CLAUSE

(A) *I nominate, constitute and appoint my spouse, Nil, and my oldest sister, Njeri, to be the Executors of my estate.*

(B) *If, for any reason, my first nominees Executors should fail to qualify or be unable or unwilling to accept or to continue as the Executors of my Estate, I nominate, constitute and appoint my friends James and Shandra to be Executors of my Estate.*

EXECUTOR POWER OF APPOINTMENT CLAUSE

(A) *All directives in this Will that use by reference the word Executor mean and include any person named herein as my Executor (or personal representative, as may be defined under state law) and any person who may be acting in either capacity, at any time. Such person shall have broad and reasonable discretion under the directives of this my Last Will and Testament with respect to any personal property left or held by me.*

(B) *I wish my Executors to have a broad and reasonable discretion in administration of my property, to have all powers permitted to be exercised by an Executor under state law, and to be able to do anything they deem advisable for the best interest of all without the necessity of court approval or supervision. I direct my Executors perform all acts, take all such proceedings, and exercises all such rights and privileges, although not specifically mentioned in this Will, with relation to any such property, as if the absolute owner thereof; and in connection therewith, to make, execute and deliver any instruments, and to enter into any covenants or agreements binding my Estate or any portion thereof.*

(C) *No such person named in, or appointed in connection with this Will in a fiduciary capacity shall be required to file any bond or other security for the faithful performance of his or her duties as such fiduciary in any jurisdiction, and if, despite this directive, a bond should be required, I request that it be accepted without sureties and in a nominal amount.*

SAVING CLAUSE

If a court of competent jurisdiction shall at any time invalidate or find unenforceable any provision of this Will, such invalidation shall not be construed as invalidating the whole Will. All of the remaining provisions shall be undisturbed as to their legal force and effect. If a court finds that an invalidated or unenforceable provision would become valid if it is limited, then such provision shall be deemed to be written, construed and enforced as so limited.

IN WITNESS WHEREOF, *the undersigned Testator, declare that I sign and execute this instrument of the date written below as my Last Will and Testament and further declare that I sign it willingly, that I execute it as my free and voluntary act for the purposes expressed in this document that I am eighteen years of age or older, of sound mind and under no constraint or undue influence.*

_____

(Signature of Lucy Wairimu Gathungu)

SSN:
DATE:

ATTESTATION CLAUSE

This Last Will and Testament, which had been separately signed by Lucy, the Testator, was signed, executed and declared by the above named Testator as his or her Last Will and Testament in the presence of each of us. We, in the presence of the Testator and each other, under penalty of perjury, hereby subscribe our names as witnesses to the declaration and execution of the Last Will and Testament by the Testator, and we declare that, to the best of our knowledge, said Testator is eighteen years of age or older, of sound mind and under no constraint or undue influence.

1. _____   _____
   (Signature of Witness)   *(Print Name)*
   Date: _____   _____
                                      (Address)

                                      _____
                                      (City, State, Zip)

2. _____   _____
   (Signature of Witness)   *(Print Name)*
   Date: _____   _____
                                      (Address)

                                      _____
                                      (City, State, Zip)

STATEMENT OF INTERMENT, CREMATION AND WISHES

I, Lucy Wairimu Gathungu, the undersigned, having previously executed a Last Will and Testament of the date hereof, hereby state that, in addition to the directives bequests set forth in said Last Will and Testament, is my desire that my remains be interred in my parents' farm in Kenya.

My further wishes and directives are as follows: I would like to have a Christian burial. I would like a Christian service in Virginia to celebrate my life before making the final journey home to Kenya. I would like everyone to know that I thank God for all the blessings in my life. To my husband, Nil, my parents,

John and Esther Gathungu, my sisters, Njeri, Gloria, Lydiah, Nancy, my brother, Jeff, my nieces Julie, Nina, Ethel, Jazmine, my nephews Richard (Koki), Waititu, Ian, Ethan, Eli, Ezekiel, my "grandchildren" Nisey and Jude, my in-laws, my relatives, my friends and my wonderful medical team, I love you and I will see you again in heaven. May God be with you.

Dated: _____

_____

(Signature of Lucy Wairimu Gathungu)

WITNESS ATTESTATION CLAUSE

This statement of interment, Cremation and Wishes, which has been separately signed by Lucy W. Gathungu was signed, executed and declared in the presence of each of us. We, in the presence of Lucy W. Gathungu and each other, under penalty of perjury, hereby subscribe our names as witnesses to the declaration and execution of the Statement of Interment, Cremation and Wishes by Lucy W. Gathungu and we declare that, to the best of our knowledge, Lucy is eighteen years of age or older, of sound mind and under no constraint or undue influence.

1. _____   _____
   (Signature of Witness)   *(Print Name)*
   Date: _____   _____
                                      (Address)

                                      _____
                                      (City, State, Zip)

2. _____   _____
   (Signature of Witness)   *(Print Name)*
   Date: _____   _____
                                      (Address)

                                      _____
                                      (City, State, Zip)

SELF-PROVING AFFIDAVIT

Commonwealth of Virginia

County of _____

    I, Lucy Wairimu Gathungu, the undersigned Testator, being first duly sworn, do declare to the undersigned authority that I signed and executed the attached or annexed instruments as my Last Will and Testament and that I signed it willingly, that I executed it as my free and voluntary act for the purposes expressed in that document and that at the time I signed the document, I was eighteen years or older, of sound mind and under no constraint or undue influence.

Date: _____

_____

(Signature of Lucy Wairimu Gathungu)

We, the undersigned witnesses, being first duly sworn, do each declare to the undersigned authority the following: (1) the Testator declared to each of us that the attached or annexed instrument of his or her Last Will and Testament; (2)the Testator executed the will in our presence;(3) each of us in the presence of the Testator, signed the will as witness, and (4) to the best of our knowledge, the Testator is eighteen years of age or older, of sound mind and under no constraint or undue influence.

_____   _____

(Signature of Witness)   (Print Name)

_____   _____

(Signature of Witness)   (Print Name)

<u>Acknowledgment of Notary Public:</u>

Subscribed, sworn and acknowledged to me on this _____day of _____20____, by Lucy Wairimu Gathungu as Testator, and _____and _____ _____as witnesses.

Witness my hand seal.

Signature of Notary Public: _____

The witnesses and the notary left after about twenty minutes, and Njeri returned to the room. Lucy handed Njeri the papers and asked that she keeps them with her at all times. She called the attending head nurse and gave her the power of attorney, appointing Njeri as her spokesperson in case she became unable to speak for herself.

"Now, I can have peace, knowing that Nil will not try to deny Mami and Baba the right to say good-bye to their child," Lucy said before falling into a long, deep sleep.

CHAPTER 17

Be True to Yourself

As one would expect, Lucy was tired of the hospital room. Each day she was hopeful that it would be the day that she would finally have a bowel movement so the doctors could send her home. Although the doctors had told her that the cancer was terminal, Lucy hung on to the slim chance that chemo might shrink the tumors in her colon. Lucy didn't eat by mouth for almost two weeks. Instead, she received tube feeding, through her arm, a process called parenteral nutrition (PN). The doctors, nurses, and dieticians were frequently monitoring her potassium, sugar, and sodium to make sure they were not at dangerous levels. Lucy would crave certain foods and thought it wouldn't hurt to ask.

"I know I can't have anything solid to eat, but what if I have the food pureed?" Lucy asked one of the doctors.

"If you can have it pureed to very fine consistency, like a milk shake, then you can have a small amount," the doctor responded.

This made Lucy happy; the first thing she craved was Kenya chai.

One evening when Njeri was spending the night, Lucy said that she felt terrible that she had so many unanswered calls because it was hard for her to speak with the NG tube. Njeri suggested they create a central place where only friends and family could visit for updates using CaringBridge.org; Lucy agreed to do so, and Njeri started the page.

As Lucy had requested, Njeri and Gloria brought in Ethel, Jazmine, and Ian to visit her one evening. The girls had created a collage of photographs of all Lucy's nieces, nephews, and great-nieces and great-nephews on a poster.

Lucy was so touched by the poster that she asked the girls to hang it over Nil's schedule in order to obscure it.

"Ian, did you bring me what I asked you?" Lucy asked her nephew. Ian gave Lucy a small bag of fries.

"You can't have those," Gloria said.

"Watch me," Lucy said as she took one French fry from the small bag. "I only want the taste. I'll spit it out." Lucy slowly chewed the French fry, asked for a napkin, and spit it out. She did this a couple of times, then announced that the craving was over. She told the children she wanted to tell them something important and to pay attention. The children quietly sat around the small bed, and Lucy started to speak.

"You are not babies anymore, so I know you are well aware of what's going on. The doctors have said that I don't have long to live; I personally think they are wrong, but if this is it, I want you to know how much I love you. I have always thought of you and your cousins in Kenya as my own children. I have enjoyed seeing you grow to become the awesome people you are. I am very proud of you.

"I hope that once you are ready to find mates, you will find people that love and care about you. Don't rush into marriage, especially if you have a bad feeling about it. Remember what Maya Angelou says, 'When someone shows you who they are, believe them.' If someone shows you their crazy side, you'd better believe that's who they are. Don't think you can change a grown man or woman, and also, do not make a mistake of falling for someone who wants to keep you for themselves; that is not love. That is control. Don't tell yourself lies; always be true to yourself.

"Education is important because it allows you to be independent. Always try to learn something new, whatever it may be. Always strive to better yourself, no matter what the circumstances are. Have goals in life, even when they seem impossible, and slowly work toward them.

"The best gift Mami and Baba gave me is faith. Without it, I don't know how I would have survived all that I have been through. Find something to believe in; start by reading the Bible every day and meditate on it. Don't let people interpret it for you; ask questions and strive to get answers. Start your day with gratitude, remembering that there are many who would have loved to be alive on this particular day, but did not live to see it. Remember, it feels better to give than to receive so, please, find a way to give back in whichever way you can.

"Most importantly, as Mami says, love your family. When all is said and done, your family will stick by you. Never, ever let anyone come between you and the family. Our family is tight. Let's keep it that way. I need to stop talking now. Ian, give me another French fry!"

Lucy eyes were tearing up; she sat up to go to the bathroom. Njeri turned off the suction device and disconnected the collector. When Lucy returned, Njeri reconnected and turned on the suction tube and then lengthened the tube to let the contents flow into the collector. "Oh my God, look, there is a small piece of French fry in there," Lucy said, laughing loudly. "I thought I chewed it enough."

"You were not supposed to swallow it, Aunty Lucy. You said you would spit it all out," Ian said.

"Oh well, I am busted," Lucy said and got back in bed. "I love you guys; you should go. It's almost ten p.m. Gloria, I am worried about the condition of your car. You should take mine, since I am not using it, so you can come to see me whenever you are free without worrying that you will break down."

"It's too costly to get the car fixed now, but I will get it done next month," Gloria said. "Yes, I could be here often if we had two cars, but no worries."

"My car is not being used. So take the keys so when Ian goes to school tomorrow, you can come over," Lucy said.

"I'll take the keys another day, sis. I'll drop Ian off to school, and then I'll be here early tomorrow. Good night," Gloria said as she left the room. The children hugged Njeri and Lucy and followed Gloria out of the room. Lucy was scheduled to have chemo the following morning.

CHAPTER 18

Caring and Compassion

LUCY RECEIVED HER LAST CHEMO treatment on Wednesday, August 27, 2016. When she walked into the treatment room to prep for chemo, she caught a glimpse of a former coworker who had recently been diagnosed with breast cancer. Lucy hugged the lady tightly; they were both sobbing. They wished each other well, and then Lucy sat on her chair as she had done more times than she could now count. Gloria stayed with her during this chemo.

After chemo, Lucy and Gloria returned to the room where again, Lucy was hooked up to the machines that were helping her. Njeri stayed with her that night, and for the first time, she understood what Lucy meant when she said she couldn't sleep after chemo. They stayed up all night, walking through the halls of the hospital. Lucy did most of the talking, telling Njeri about the book she was writing. Lucy felt lucky that she was surrounded by loving and caring people. She was humbled that so many cared about her. Her phone rang constantly; she was receiving well wishes on her CaringBridge webpage, and there was no shortage of visitors in her room.

Lucy looked forward to the visits from her friends. She laughed and joked with her "sister friends" Tamara, Diane, Pauline, Shandra, and Tina. She found it hard to believe that some colleagues at the Dumfries Health Center took time out of their busy schedules to visit with her. Her friend Tina organized a "Lucy's day" and collected cards with well wishes. Two of Fort Belvoir's clergy, Reverend Father Opara and Chaplain(MAJ) Nobles, visited Lucy every weekday and sometimes on the weekend. They prayed with her, encouraged her, and read the scriptures with her. Lucy talked to them freely, and each time they left her room, she felt hopeful that indeed, God had not abandoned her. Lucy grew very fond of her chemo nurse, Anita, who introduced Lucy to her pastors, Jonathan and Quanetta Lewis. These two pastors adopted Lucy as though she were their church member. They stopped by most evenings to sit with her, talk to her, and share God's word with her.

Lucy was getting a lot of attention from the staff at Fort Belvoir; they would come into the room to talk to her. Lucy would ask them about their families and listened intently as they talked at length. Every other day, the massage therapist, Ms. Elizabeth, would stop by to give Lucy a full-body massage, something that Lucy looked forward to. There was also the doctor who would massage her stomach, gently following her colon track to ease some of the discomfort and perhaps trigger a bowel movement. Lucy was grateful for all this.

Nil, too, brought well wishes from his work colleagues. He walked into the hospital room one day and showed Lucy a few get well soon cards with gift cards in them. He left the room only to return a couple of hours later with thank-you cards. He couldn't find the gift cards and accused Njeri and Lucy of taking them.

"Are you crazy. What would I do with gift cards?" Lucy asked him.

"I left them here. They didn't walk off by themselves," Nil replied sarcastically. After, he searched his bag frantically, he found the cards. He wrote the thank-you cards, sealed each envelop, then left the room, making sure he did not leave the cards behind.

"He is so uncouth," Lucy said. "What the heck was I thinking? Love is truly blind."

"You still love him, don't you, sis?" Njeri asked.

"I love him as a human being; how can I hate him? I believe God used him as a vehicle so I can get these great doctors. I have forgiven him for his stupidity."

CHAPTER 19

Double Trouble

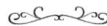

NIL AVOIDED THE HOSPITAL WHENEVER the sisters were with Lucy. Whenever he walked in and found them, he would ask them to leave so he could be alone with his wife. The sisters would only return when he left, which was never long. Lucy would be upset whenever he came because all he wanted was for her to sign papers agreeing to give him the power of attorney and the right to bury her. He told Lucy that he had spoken to the lawyers and they would be calling her to verify if she wanted their service.

Early one morning, Lucy received a call from the military lawyer Nil had spoken to. When the lawyer asked Lucy if she wanted him to come to the room to sign papers, Lucy said she had signed all the papers she was going to sign. The lawyer advised Lucy not to sign anything that she was not comfortable signing. Nil was livid when he found out that Lucy refused to sign his papers. He came into the hospital room that afternoon and asked to speak to Njeri outside. Lucy gave an agreeable nod, and Njeri stepped out with Nil.

"Ya'll refuse to plan Lucy's funeral, so I will go ahead and plan it by myself," Nil said, staring intently at Njeri. "Ya'll in denial, but I gotta do what I gotta do. Lucy is my wife whether ya'll like it or not. She is my responsibility, and I don't care what ya'll do. I gotta take care of business."

"Lucy is still here, Nil. She does not want to discuss her funeral. She is not stupid. She is well aware of her mortality. In my culture, we do not bury people before they are dead. Lucy does not wish to discuss her funeral plans, and I respect that. I think you should, too," Njeri responded.

"Like I said, I will do what I gotta do. If ya'll want your parents to come for the funeral, then ya'll better make arrangements," Nil said nonchalantly.

"Lucy told me that she has emphatically told you that she wishes to be buried next to my sister in Kenya. You refuse to acknowledge that and keep pestering her. Who does that? I don't think you care what happens. You just want to get it over with." Njeri's voice was shaking with emotion.

"Who do you think you are talking to?" Nil retorted. "I don't want you visiting my wife anymore. I don't want you or your sisters here anymore."

"Nil, first of all, Lucy is my baby sister, so there is nothing you can do to keep me away from her. Second, my husband is retired from the military, and I have a military ID; so I can come in and out of Fort Belvoir as I please. You are out of your mind. It will take the military police to kick me out of here. I am not going anywhere. You can go if you want to."

"Fuck you," Nil said as he walked away.

Njeri returned to the room to find Lucy anxious to know what had transpired. She told Lucy that Nil wanted to discuss funeral plans, to which she responded, "I was going to mention my will to him, but I won't waste my time. *Ngoma ni itwo ngoma.*" (Call out on evil.)

"Let's not waste our time talking about him anymore," Njeri said.

Later that day, Nil walked into the room accompanied by one of his older sisters, Luna. Njeri was sitting by the window, going through her e-mails as Lucy was sleeping. Luna said hello and proceeded to wake Lucy up. Nil ignored Njeri.

Due to constant pain, Lucy was connected intravenously to the patient-controlled analgesia pump (PAC), which allowed her to deliver her own pain medication whenever she needed it. Every time she did this, she would fall into a deep sleep. Nil and Luna walked in soon after Lucy had pressed the PAC, so she woke up groggy, said a quick hello, and fell right back to sleep.

Njeri sat silently as Luna kept trying to wake Lucy up but finally said, "Maybe you should give her time to sleep the medicine off; she will wake up soon."

This remark irritated Nil, and he told his sister how Njeri thought she made decisions around the hospital. Njeri was silent because she did not want a repeat of what had transpired earlier that morning between her and Nil.

"How would you feel if this were your husband, what's his name?" Luna asked Njeri.

"My husband's name is Tony, but I don't know what you are asking," Njeri replied.

"How would you feel if Tony was lying in bed dying and his sisters or brothers were taking over the show and not allowing you to make plans for his funeral?" Luna asked.

"I can assure you that I would honor my husband's wishes, and he would honor mine, too," Njeri responded.

"When two people get married, they should be left alone. You should stay out of Nil and Lucy's business," Luna said.

"Lucy comes from a close family. Our culture does not call for family to abandon a sick loved one so I am here to support my sister as long as she needs me."

"You are in America now, so fuck your culture. Lucy is my wife," Nil jumped in.

"And I am here to support my brother. He called me to come and help him, and I am here," Luna said, discharging saliva as she spoke.

"I will not have an argument with you guys. I do not wish to speak to either of you from here on. Do what you feel you must," Njeri said as she walked out of the room.

Shortly after Njeri left, Nil and Luna left the room and ignored Njeri, who was in the waiting room. Njeri walked back to Lucy's room and found her sitting up, sipping a glass of ice water.

"I heard everything, sis. I am so sorry; I never imagined it would come to this. I am going to call Nil's sisters who are sensible and ask them to talk to Luna. She is so shameless; walking in here and instead of asking how I am doing, she attacks you. She is jealous that my family cares about me. She doesn't talk to her own children and does not get along with the rest of the family. Evil has a twin sister, and her name is Luna."

"Don't worry, sis. I am a big girl. Everything they say bounces off me and sticks to them," Njeri said, smiling.

"The pain is getting intense again, so I will push the PAC and go back to sleep. Are you spending the night today?"

"Gloria is coming to spend the night, sis. I'll wait until she gets here."

Gloria was on her way to the hospital when she received a call from Nil. At first, she thought something had happened to Lucy because Nil never called her. "I hear you are planning on driving Lucy's car. Don't even think about it," Nil said and hung up the phone.

Njeri arrived early the following morning to relieve Gloria who had to go to work that afternoon. Gloria had made Lucy her morning chai, which Lucy sipped on. Lately, she could only take a couple of sips. Lydiah called, as she did every morning, to talk to Lucy, who wanted to know what her three nephews were up to. Lucy also spoke to Mami and Baba, as she did every day, reassuring them that she was doing well under the circumstances. This morning, Lucy was in a joking mood as she spoke to her parents.

"Baba, do you have pocket money?" she asked in Kikuyu. "You know, you cannot go around town with nothing in your pockets yet tell folks that your children in America are doing great. I will send you some pocket money."

The good mood was short-lived as Nil and Luna walked in that afternoon with a folder and propped it in Lucy's sight.

"I want to talk to my wife alone," Nil said.

"I want Njeri to stay here. What is it, Nil?" Lucy asked.

"Now I can't talk to you?"

Njeri was afraid of where this conversation was going so she left the room only to be followed by Luna. They sat on opposite sides of the sides of the waiting room. Shortly after, Shandra followed by Tina came by to visit Lucy. Shandra, who had met Luna before, said hello.

"People need to mind their own business. People shouldn't mess around with married folks. My brother called me, and I am here to support him. I don't care if no one talks to me," Luna told Shandra. Njeri walked away and returned only after she saw Luna and Nil leaving the hospital.

"She came here with guns blazing and ready to fight you," Shandra told Njeri as they walked to Lucy's room.

"I could not care less," Njeri said.

"Luna and Nil finalized my funeral plans today. He wanted me to see the folder," Lucy said quietly after Tina and Shandra left.

CHAPTER 20

All I Want Is Peace

Ms. Donna had been Lucy's social worker for a few years, and they had grown fond of each other. Ms. Donna visited Lucy every day during the week unless she was out of the office. Their conversations were private, and neither Nil or Njeri were allowed to attend the sessions. Following Luna's departure, Ms. Donna approached Njeri and asked if she would be willing to meet with Nil and Lucy to figure out how to move forward. She said that if Njeri were willing, she would ask Nil if he, too, was willing. Njeri agreed.

Nil was in the room when Njeri arrived at the hospital at the set time. She waited outside for Ms. Donna to arrive. They walked in together; Njeri knew that Lucy was nervous about the meeting. She hugged her and whispered in her ear in Swahili, *"Usijali, Siste. Kila kitu poa,"* meaning, "Don't worry, sis. Everything is fine."

"I wanted to meet both of you because Lucy wishes that you two would get along," Ms. Donna started. "I ask that we all listen to one another without interrupting. Lucy, can you tell them what you told me?"

"I just want peace. Nil, I always tell you that I love you no matter what. You know things haven't been good between us. I always hoped that this marriage would work, but it hasn't. I love my sisters, and I can't imagine what life would be like without them. I am tired of you going off on my sisters. I know I am legally your wife, but this is my family, and I need them around me." Two big teardrops rolled down Lucy's face.

"Lucy told me that you've each said things to each other in the heat of the moment. Njeri, can I ask you, did you mean what you said when you are angry?"

"I did not mean the things said in anger, and I apologize," Njeri said.

"What about you, Nil? Did you mean the things you said in anger?"

"Yes, I did. I meant every word I said. They refuse to discuss Lucy's funeral plans."

"I already told you that I want to be buried in Kenya, at my parents' farm next to my sister Shiku," Lucy said.

"That's not going to happen. It will be too expensive," Nil said.

"I told you that Njeri will take care of it. She can help navigate the process. Kenyans do this all the time."

"How do we move forward? Lucy, do you feel like you are being forced to choose between your family and your husband?"

"Nil is unreasonable by expecting my family to stay away from me. Nil, you know I like it when you give me attention and spoil me, but this is my family. I told you a long time ago that my family is important to me," Lucy said.

"I love my sister," Njeri started. "A long time ago, I read a play called the *Caucasian Chalk Circle* where two women went to court to claim a child they each believed rightfully belongs to them. After hearing the argument, the judge orders a chalk circle to be drawn and places the child in the middle. He then orders the women to pull the child and whoever wins takes the child. One woman refuses to pull; I, too, refuse to pull. I am willing to do whatever Nil is asking within reason. We gave him a schedule, but he doesn't communicate what he wants from us."

"Is that OK with you, Nil? Can you communicate better on what you expect the sisters to do?" Ms. Donna asked.

"I will only deal with her; I don't want to speak to the others," Nil said.

Nil started speaking to Njeri after this meeting. Lucy thought he was calmer because he had finalized the funeral plans. He told Njeri that he had rented a room at a hotel nearby and would be staying late with Lucy for the next two days. Lucy felt that if he indeed wanted to stay with her, he would not need to book a hotel room. Njeri told Lucy that she was a phone call away if Lucy needed her.

For reasons unknown to Gloria and her son, Ian, Nil was more hostile toward them. On a day that Gloria was scheduled to be at the hospital, she was running late due to car problems and getting lost after using a different gate to enter the military base. Gloria called Lucy's phone to let her know that she was running late, but Lucy did not pick up. Gloria decided to call Nil's phone, which turned out to be a big mistake. Nil told Gloria to stay where she was and he would meet her. When Gloria spotted Nil, she started driving to follow him, but he stopped, got out of the car, and headed toward her.

"What is wrong with you? You said you would be here in the morning, and you were not," Nil yelled at Gloria.

"I am sorry. I am having car trouble. Ian and I came here as fast as we could," Gloria responded.

"Ya'll think you can do whatever you want. I've been trying to talk to you about Lucy's funeral plans, but you keep ignoring me. I don't care what ya'll think. I am going to have her cremated," Nil said.

"I don't know why you are yelling at me, and Lucy does not wish to be cremated," Gloria responded.

Nil continued yelling at Gloria. Ian held his mother's hand and said, *"Mum, wachana nayeye, twende,"* meaning, "Mum, leave him alone, and let's go." Ian got into the driver's seat. Nil got into his car and drove off; Ian followed him, hoping he was going in the direction of the hospital.

Gloria did not want to stress Lucy by telling her about what had transpired between her and Nil. She called Njeri, obviously upset.

"Sis, his yelling came out of nowhere. I didn't do anything to trigger him but call to let him know I was lost and I was running late," Gloria said.

"It's not your fault. He is obviously projecting his anger toward you. We should feel sorry for him. As Lucy says, 'Forgive him.'" Njeri tried to console her sister.

"He said he had decided to have Lucy cremated. There is nothing wrong with cremation, but that is not what Lucy wants. How can he plan to go against her wishes? I am going in to see Lucy, and I don't want her to see me crying. Ian is there with her now. I will get something to drink, then go into the room. Love you, sis. I am OK. I have bigger fish to fry instead of being upset by a nincompoop, as Baba would say," Gloria told Njeri before hanging up the phone.

The chemo side effects were long gone, but the pain had become more intense for Lucy. She was concerned that the chemo had not shrunk the tumors enough, as she was yet to have a bowel movement. As the days went by, her hands started shaking whenever she was in severe pain. She was also getting a back injection that raised her blood pressure every time the nurse came into the room to administer it. The only nurse that Lucy thought was doing it right was Ms. May; this was because she had Lucy take deep breaths and hold one of her sisters' or whoever was in the room's hands as she administered the injection. Lydiah came over for the weekend as she always did and spend the night with Lucy, chatting late into the night. Gloria and Ian stopped by in the evening, and Lucy wouldn't stop telling funny stories, even getting out of the bed to make fun of Njeri's dancing moves.

Lucy was nostalgic about the days she used to go to the gym, so she asked one of the doctors if she could go. She asked Njeri to bring her sweatpants and a T-shirt to wear to the gym. On September 1, 2014, the doctor took her to the gym, and Lucy exercised for a short while before the pain took over. The doctor was impressed and told the sisters what a remarkable woman Lucy was. That same day, Lucy's favorite of Nil's sisters, Joy, and her husband came to visit, which made Lucy very happy. On September 3, the doctors told the family that they would discharge Lucy to get home care through hospice. Lucy was not fond of the word *hospice* because she thought it implied that the hospital could do nothing else for her. She asked her sisters not to use the name hospice because it made her sad, but instead use the term home care.

As it turned out, Lucy would not leave the hospital.

CHAPTER 21

The Last Days

ARRANGEMENTS FOR LUCY TO RECEIVE care at her home stalled when the hospital staff found out that Nil had stopped paying into the secondary Medicare insurance that Lucy had qualified for after she stopped working. It was challenging finding a homecare service that took military insurance alone. The nurse leading the effort to get Lucy's coverage was Ms. John. She spent many hours working on the case and, eventually, found a company that would suffice.

Ms. John went into Lucy's room to give her the good news. Lucy was happy that she was leaving the hospital but concerned that Nil would make it difficult for her sisters to come in to see her. Ms. John asked if Lucy would rather go to Njeri's house, and Lucy said she would consider it. Ms. John talked to the social worker, Ms. Donna, about Lucy's concern. The doctors, Ms. John, and Ms. Donna agreed to add a condition that Nil must allow Lucy's sisters to care for her. Lucy was scheduled to leave the hospital for home care on Friday, September 5, 2014.

Nil told the sisters that he would stay on Wednesday night. When Njeri and Gloria came to see Lucy on Thursday morning, Lucy told them that she no longer wanted Nil to stay with her. She told them that all he did was complain and ask why bad things happened to him. She also told them that he kept getting phone calls and stepping out to answer them and she knew they were from Yanna. At some point, Nil had left the room, and Lucy had spent most of the night alone except for the staff that occasionally stopped in the room to take her vitals and medicate her. Lucy couldn't sleep, so she had spent the waking hours making a necklace for her chemo nurse, Anita. She was proud of the fact that she had completed this task even with shaky hands. She proudly gave Anita the necklace when she came to visit her that morning, then went right back to sleep.

Anita and Njeri were sitting quietly in the room when two nurses walked in to change the NG tube. For the first time, Lucy cried as they did it. "Everything hurts. I don't want to die," she kept repeating.

Njeri was hugging her tightly and said the first thing that came to mind. "Believers don't die, sis. They go to heaven to be with Jesus."

Anita could not hold her tears; she gave Lucy a hug, whispered, "I love you," and left the room. It would be the last time Anita saw Lucy alive.

When the clergy came to visit, Lucy told them that she thought she would die soon. She seemed resigned that this indeed was the end. The pain was intolerable, and the PCA pump did not give her much relief. The nurses came in more often to give her medication to ease the pain.

"I want you to stay with me no matter what Nil says or does," Lucy told Njeri.

Njeri could not fall asleep on Thursday night. She took Lucy's iPad and Googled Kikuyu and Swahili songs they had known as children and sang them softly. After a while Lucy joined her, singing what she remembered. They started taking turns on song selection, and to their surprise, they found them all, even some on YouTube. Lucy asked Njeri to continue singing because her throat felt irritated.

Before sending Lucy home, the attending physician ordered a variety of tests. The results showed that her blood levels were very low, and she required a transfusion. Njeri called to let Nil know that Lucy would not be released that day. He told Njeri that the home care people had delivered a bed and set it up for Lucy. Nil said he would come by the hospital so Njeri could go home. Lucy was quiet the entire morning but would ask Njeri how she was doing whenever she woke up to get her pain medication.

Nil came in that afternoon and said he would spend the night. Njeri asked him politely if she could spend the night with Lucy. "She likes me to sing to her," Njeri said. "I really would appreciate if you allow me to spend the night with her again today, please," she begged, and Nil agreed.

Njeri returned to Fort Belvoir hospital after 6:00 p.m. Nil was sitting on a chair in the room, surfing the web. The curtains in the room were drawn; it was very dark except for a dim light on Lucy's bedside.

"She had some type of bowel movement," Nil told Njeri as he put his put his laptop in its case.

Shortly after midnight on Friday, September 5, 2014, the nurse walked into the room to take Lucy's vitals and noticed that her oxygen level was low and her blood pressure very high. A few minutes later, there was a team of doctors in the room examining her. Njeri left the room, nervously shaking, not wanting Lucy to see that she was deathly scared. After composing herself, she walked in to find Lucy laughing, telling the doctors that it tickled when they touched her stomach. At 1:00 a.m., a decision was made to take her into ICU so they could monitor her more closely.

As Lucy was being wheeled away, she called out to her sister, "Njeri, grab my iPhone and keep it with you no matter what." Njeri saw the pink-cased iPhone next to the bed, picked it up, and put it her pocket.

Njeri called Nil to let him know that Lucy was going into ICU. "I know I shouldn't have left," Nil said.

He arrived at the ICU with a suitcase and talked to the doctor in charge. Whatever he was told made him angry, and he demanded that everyone leave the ICU room so he could speak to his wife alone. Nil then walked to the room where Lucy had stayed for three weeks, packed everything in the suitcase, including her journals, her laptop, her iPad, her clothes, and everything else he felt was of value. He left the cards, plants, and flowers that Lucy's friends and family had brought to her over the course of the hospital stay. At that point, Nil would not return to the hospital even after getting multiple calls from the emergency room doctors, as he was still the next of kin. Fortunately, Lucy had not only told Njeri she was ready but had also given her the power of attorney, so when the doctors informed her that there was nothing else they could do for Lucy, Njeri consulted with her sisters, and together, they told the doctors to make Lucy comfortable. For two and a half hours, they sang hymns, prayed, and read passages from the Bible. At 12:10 p.m., Lucy passed away, peacefully, surrounded by people who loved her.

CHAPTER 22
What Now?

THE ICU DOCTOR CAME INTO the room to let the family know that Lucy had died. Even though they had all watched as Lucy gasped three times for air and Gloria had said it was done, the machines were still active, and Njeri wasn't sure that indeed Lucy was gone. The doctor hugged everyone, then left the room. The chaplain said a prayer, and then they all walked into the waiting room. The doctor called Njeri aside to ask if she wanted to get an autopsy done. He explained that if this was requested, they would not unhook Lucy from the machines. The doctor also told Njeri that they had called Nil to tell him that Lucy had died. Njeri told the doctors that it would be best to wait for Nil to see what he wanted to do. The doctor explained that under the directive Lucy had provided, Njeri was legally the person who could make the call. Njeri asked the doctor what was next. The doctor said he would call someone to come and talk to the family.

While they sat in the waiting room, Njeri mentioned to James for the first time that Lucy had a will. She handed the will to James, who read through it.

"You may need a lawyer," he said.

They sat quietly in the waiting room; the children who had been kept away from the ICU looked confused. Lydiah suggested that her husband Mike and Ian to go to Njeri's house and wait. Njeri, Lydiah, and Gloria were alone in the waiting room when a young, uniformed female soldier and a middle-aged-looking female hospital administrator walked into the room and introduced themselves.

"I am very sorry for the loss," the soldier started; the same was echoed by the administrator.

"Thank you. What should we expect next?" Njeri asked.

"Today is Saturday, so your sister will be taken to the morgue and will not be transferred until Monday," the soldier said.

"My sister's wishes were to be buried in Kenya, but we know that her husband does not agree," Gloria said. "Is there anyone we can present her will to here at the hospital?"

"I am sorry, but her husband is the next of kin, so whatever he decides to do will be final," the soldier responded.

"That is not fair. There has to be a way that someone can look at the will to see my sister's wish." Lydiah jumped in.

"Well, for now, he has the right to get the body. Maybe eventually you can go to court to have the body exhumed so you can take your sister to Nigeria."

The sisters could not believe what this young woman was saying; they didn't try to correct her assumption that they wanted to take Lucy's remains to Nigeria. The hospital administrator interrupted the soldier and said that they did not have the answer to the question and that the sisters would have to wait until Monday to talk to others who may know the answers, including the military law office.

Nil, his sister Joy, and her husband and their friend walked into the waiting room soon after the soldier and administrator had left. Joy hugged the sisters, telling them how sorry she was. Her husband and friend did the same. Nil stood in the other corner of the room without saying a word. Njeri asked him if he wished to have an autopsy done and he loudly said no. Unbeknownst to the sisters, the four had already gone into the ICU room to see Lucy.

"What do we do now? Will you honor Lucy's wishes?" Njeri asked Nil.

"I tried to talk to ya'll, but you refused. I have already made plans," Nil said.

"What plans did you make?" Njeri asked quietly.

"I will have her taken to the funeral home on Monday morning."

"What funeral home?"

"A. L. Bennett and Son Funeral Home in Fredericksburg, Virginia, "Nil responded, then said, "Joy, let's get out of here."

"We will make the funeral arrangements. You do not have to do anything. If you want to be included in the obituary, you will have to give Nil your names, including your parents' names," Joy said.

The sisters looked at one another in disbelief. Lydiah's face indicated she was ready to pounce; Njeri and Gloria knew something was about to happen, so they managed to get Lydiah out of the room. The sisters were left in the room alone until the staff from the sixth floor brought them the flowers and cards that Nil had left behind. They all had great things to say about Lucy, especially her sense of humor. They seemed shocked that she had died.

The ICU nurse came into the waiting room to tell the sisters that she had removed the tubes from Lucy's face. When the three walked into the room, they stopped in their tracks. Lying on the bed with two pillows propping her head was Lucy. Her black, shiny, thick, curly hair looked as though she had just styled it. Her face was relaxed and glowing as though she had applied a small amount of skin foundation. Her lips were slightly parted, giving the appearance of a smile.

"She died smiling," Gloria said.

"I haven't seen her relaxed in years," Njeri said.

"She now has the peace she wanted, finally," Lydiah said.

The sisters each kissed Lucy, talking to her as though she could hear. They went back to the waiting room and called Mami, Baba, and family members. Njeri looked through Lucy's phone, and together, they called Lucy's close friends to let them know she had died. They did not want family and friends to find out about Lucy's death on Facebook. Afterward, the sisters carried the flowers and plants to the car and drove silently to Njeri's house where the rest of the family had gathered.

CHAPTER 23

Family, Friends, and the Kenyan Diaspora

ALTHOUGH THE SISTERS HAD WITNESSED Lucy's death, there was still a strong sense of disbelief. It all seemed like a bad dream from which they would all wake. The constant ringing of their cell phones reminded the sisters that, indeed, Lucy was gone. Njeri, Gloria, Lydiah, and their families knew they had to act quickly to make sure that Lucy's wishes were honored. James and Tony suggested that they find a lawyer before the weekend was over.

The family needed help from their Kenyan friends who were familiar with transporting remains outside the United States. First, Njeri called her longtime friend Sang, who was an active member of the Kenyan Diaspora. Njeri was sure that Sang could provide guidance, as he had sadly experienced the loss of his wife, Maureen, and taken her body to Kenya for burial. Njeri received calls from other longtime friends, Rachel, Fred, Pam, Rae, and Sonya, all pledging support and giving great advice. Gloria and Lydiah received calls from their friends, too. Within three hours, Sang and Pam were at Njeri's house. Sang read Lucy's will and agreed with Tony that the family needed to get a lawyer as soon as possible. Another friend, Frank, heard the news of Lucy's death from Dr. Githaiga in Kenya and called Njeri immediately; after Njeri explained the dilemma, Frank provided a lawyer's name, Ms. Boyd, who he said specialized in last wills and testament. Family friends Tamara, Diane, Tina, Charlene, and their family members came to the house with food before the day was over.

One of Njeri's nephews, Tony Warui, who was in Atlanta, called a friend in Richmond, Virginia, letting him know that his aunt Lucy, a Kenyan, had passed away in Stafford. His friend called a Kenyan woman, Loyce, who lived in Stafford who immediately reached out to all the Kenyans she knew in the area. Samuel, a Kenyan colleague who had worked with Lucy at Dumfries Health Center, also sent out calls to Kenyans living in northern Virginia. That Sunday afternoon, following Lucy's death on Saturday, there was only standing room in Njeri's house. It was amazing how the community had come together to help one of their own. When the crowd of people left for the evening, the sisters opened the sympathy cards, and each had a check or cash. The total contribution toward Lucy's funeral on that Sunday was $4,000. The family was touched and encouraged. They agreed to consult with a lawyer first thing Monday morning.

Njeri left her house at 7:45 a.m. to pick up Gloria in order to go to the lawyer's office. They did not have an appointment, but they hoped that Ms. Boyd would take their case immediately due to the urgency of the situation. Njeri was distracted by her thoughts so much that she did not notice that she was driving over the limit in a school zone. A police officer stopped her and walked to her window.

"Do you know how fast you were going?" he asked.

"I am so sorry, sir. I was not paying attention. I apologize," Njeri said.

"That is a lame excuse. Give me your driver's license," the policeman said.

Njeri grabbed her purse from the passenger's seat, removed her driver's license, and handed it to the officer, who walked back to his car and returned to find Njeri drenched in tears.

"I am so sorry, Officer. I feel terrible. What if I had hit a child walking to school? It would only have complicated life. I lost my sister on Saturday, and I am distracted; this tells me I need to be more focused," Njeri cried.

The officer looked at Njeri sympathetically and said, "I am sorry for your loss. I see you have a clean driving record, so I will let you off with a warning. Pay attention when you drive. Perhaps you should not be driving." The officer handed Njeri back her license and motioned her to drive on. Njeri drove for a short distance, found a parking space in a residential neighborhood, composed herself, then continued on to Gloria's house.

They were outside the lawyer Boyd's office when they called to make an appointment. The receptionist answered the phone, saying that Ms. Boyd did not have any availability for the day. Njeri asked for just ten minutes of Ms. Boyd's time and explained the urgency. The reception put them on hold for a few minutes, then came back on the phone to ask how long it would take to get to the office. "We are outside your office. We can come in now," Njeri responded.

The receptionist walked Njeri and Gloria to a small conference room. They were soon joined by Ms. Boyd, who listened without interrupting as Njeri and Gloria told her about Lucy's life with Nil and her last will and testament, which showed that she wished to be buried in Kenya. The sisters explained that Nil had suggested cremation as an option, something Lucy did not want. Ms. Boyd looked at the will, then told the sisters that they could not expect Nil to pay for the funeral cost. The lawyer understood the urgency and agreed to take on the case. The sisters paid the retainer fee.

Ms. Boyd called the funeral home and learned that they, at Nil's request, had removed Lucy's body from Fort Belvoir to their facility early that morning. Ms. Boyd told the funeral home director that she was filing a restraining order, and they were not to do anything with Lucy's body until a decision was made in court. Within an hour, Ms. Boyd had filed a petition.

Virginia:
In the Circuit Court of Stafford County
RE: The Remains of Lucy Wairimu Gathungu
Njeri- Plaintiff v. Nil- Defendant
Petition Probate of the Estate and Restraining Order
Comes now Njeri, the oldest sister of Lucy and asks this court to allow the family to return Lucy's body to Kenya to make all funeral arrangements.

1. *Lucy was married to Nil. It was a not a happy marriage. It was an abusive one.*
2. *Lucy wrote into her Will her wishes for her body to be buried in Kenya. The will is attached as Exhibit A.*
3. *Her family is willing to pay of all expenses for carrying out her wishes, but Nil has told them he is burying her in Quantico or North Carolina.*

4. He has also told them he is going to cremate her which is against her religious beliefs.
5. Her final days were very difficult medically and Nil compounded the difficulties by being verbally abusive to her.
6. He has had numerous affairs throughout their marriage and his current girlfriend had a conversation with Lucy and told her that Nil was waiting for her to die.
7. She obliged him and passed away on Saturday, September 6, 2014.
8. The family wishes to carry out her last request to be taken home to Kenya.
9. They will pay for all the expenses of her funeral and getting her home. They fear Nil will not allow this.

NOW THEREFORE, the petitioner requests this court to issue a temporary restraining order against Nil. Specifically, that

(1) He will be enjoined from making any funeral arrangements, that her family will take care of all funeral arrangements
(2) That Nil will be enjoined from having Lucy's body cremated.
(3) That Nil will not have her buried here in the States but that Lucy's family will be permitted to return her to her home of Kenya.
(4) Any other relief the court may see fit to add.

Respectfully Requested
Njeri
By Counsel

Ms. Boyd called Njeri the next day to let her know that the court had agreed to hear the case on Wednesday, September 10, 2014. She asked that Njeri bring to court whatever evidence she had of Nil's abuse and infidelity.

Lucy had given her telephone and e-mail passwords to her sisters while she was at the hospital. Lydiah went to work to find the e-mail evidence that Lucy had talked about. Sure enough, in her Gmail account, Lucy had saved a file folder and named it "DIVORCE STUFF." Lydiah opened the folder, and in it, she found e-mail communication between Nil and his women, photographs, including one that Lucy had shown them of a woman wearing red underwear and a matching bra. Lydiah forwarded the e-mails to Njeri, who put together a package for the lawyer.

On Wednesday morning, Gloria, their friends Tamara, Donna Marie, Anita, and Pauline accompanied Njeri. Ms. Boyd showed up right before the hearing and told Njeri that Nil wanted to talk. They all walked into the courtroom to wait for the judge. Njeri sat at the front with her lawyer. Nil's lawyer sat on the other side. Nil walked in a few minutes later. He was wearing oversize Khaki pants that must have been made for a six-foot-tall man. Njeri felt sorry for him. Njeri would later learn that Nil had shown up in court wearing shorts and his lawyer had advised against it; he had borrowed the bailiff's pants. The judge came in and confirmed that both parties had agreed to discuss the matter further. She instructed that the parties return within a reasonable time to let her know if they had reached an agreement. Njeri, Ms. Boyd, Nil, and his lawyer went into a backroom office to talk.

Nil agreed to let Njeri have Lucy's body if she would cover the cost. The parties returned to the courtroom to await the judge, who said she would sign the agreement. Nil's lawyer drafted the court order:

Virginia:
In the Circuit Court of Stafford County
In re: The remains of Lucy Wairimu Gathungu
Njeri- Plaintiff v. Nil- Defendant

<u>Consent Final Order</u>
This case came this day to be heard upon the plaintiff's motion for injunction and upon the agreement of the plaintiff and defendant, as evidenced by their personal endorsements to this order, to be bound hereby and to have the rights and duties set forth herein.

Upon Consideration Whereof, it is ORDERED
1. *Pursuant to Code of Virginia section 54.1–207.01, Njeri shall have the right and the duty to direct all funeral and burial arrangements for Lucy Wairimu Gathungu. The expenses of A. L. Bennet Funeral Home through*

the entry of this order shall be borne, first by the estate of Lucy Wairimu Gathungu; and, if the estate is insufficient, by Nil. All expensed of the funeral home (and any others to carry out the rights and duties conferred upon Njeri) incurred hereafter shall be borne by Njeri. Both the plaintiff and defendant will be entitled to receive a death certificate.

2. *Nil will deliver to the office of plaintiffs' counsel in Garrisonville, Virginia, by Friday, September 12, 2014, all of the personal belongings of Lucy Wairimu Gathungu, meaning her sculptures or figurines, clothing, jewelry, Bible and passports; and Njeri shall have the right and duty (between the plaintiff and defendant) to receive them and to distribute them.*

3. *Nil will not oppose the probate of a document dated August 25, 2014, purporting to be the last will and testament of Lucy Wairimu Gathungu; and he will waive qualification as executor. He may assert allowances.*

4. *Based on the agreement of the parties and the terms of this order, the plaintiff's motion for injunction is denied. And the objects for which the suit was brought having been fully accomplished and nothing further remaining to be done herein, it is ordered that this cause be stricken from the docket and the papers placed among the ended cases, properly indexed.*

The sisters and their friends returned to Njeri's house after the hearing; they had accomplished the first step in honoring Lucy's wishes. They knew they had a steep climb ahead; they had to figure out how to raise money. Gloria and Njeri opened an account at the local bank for the purpose of keeping track of the funds. They created an account with YouCaring, the self-described compassionate crowd fund-raiser, describing Lucy's final wish to be buried in Kenya next to her sister Shiku. They had to set their grieving aside for another day and needed to focus on taking care of business at hand. Fortunately for them, they had great support from family members, friends, and the Kenyan Diaspora.

CHAPTER 24

The Spirit of Harambee

NOW THAT THE CASE HAD been settled, the funeral home had permission to make arrangements for Lucy's funeral. Njeri, Gloria, and Pauline arrived early on Thursday morning to meet the funeral director Mr. Bennett. He met them at the door, welcomed them warmly, offering his condolences, and then led them to his office. He pulled up a folder that had Lucy's name on it. He handed Njeri the itemized statement for the funeral services; it was $5,000 dollars more that the sisters had expected. Mr. Bennett explained that his funeral service had no experience shipping remains outside the United States. He would have to contract another funeral home that was familiar with the process. Njeri paid Mr. Bennett the cash she had at hand. Mr. Bennett agreed to be paid in installments. Njeri asked if they could see Lucy, to which Mr. Bennett responded that they would need time as they had not done anything to prepare her since the restraining order had been put into effect. It was agreed that the sisters would bring Lucy's clothes soon and they could visit Lucy soon after. As they were leaving the reception area to walk outside the building, Njeri, Gloria, and Pauline felt a gust of wind on their backs that stopped them in their tracks. They felt, without any doubt, that Lucy's spirit was around them.

Njeri had been having difficulty sleeping for a while. That night after the hearing, she tossed and turned for a long time, what to do next running through her mind. She remembered how caring Nil had been when Lucy was first diagnosed with colon cancer. Although it was beyond her comprehension, she knew that Lucy loved Nil, despite his infidelities and verbal abuse.

Njeri knew that Lucy would have hated seeing Nil looking so pathetic in court. Njeri remembered that Lucy had asked that she forgive Nil for all his actions. She knew she had to swallow her pride and reach out to Nil. On September 11, 2014, Njeri sent him an e-mail.

I am reaching out to you in the spirit of love, kindness, and forgiveness, which I know Lucy fully embodied. I regret that I had to file the court order, but I felt this is the only choice I had in honoring Lucy's wish to be buried in Kenya. Everyone who met Lucy knew that she truly loved you and wanted the best for you. I know, deep in my heart, her spirit wants me to come to you with an open heart.

I am including your brother, whose address I have from an e-mail you forwarded to me, in this e-mail. Our families need to support each other at this very difficult time. My mother asked me to tell you that she knows you loved Lucy and you were there for her when she needed you. I did not tell my mother I felt the need to file the order.

I believe the misunderstanding is due to our cultural differences. For Kenyans, when someone dies, families and friends make sure the funeral arrangements are taken care of. Harambee is a Kenyan tradition of community self-help events like fund-raising. Harambee literally means "all pull together" in Swahili. Many of our friends and family have pledged to help pay for Lucy's body to be transported to Kenya. Yesterday, I set up an account, and I have already started receiving funds. I will be happy to share this information with you if you are interested.

Lucy would want you to be fully engaged, so if you still want, please let's plan the Christian service in Virginia the way you think she would want it. My family and friends in Kenya will be very happy to meet and host you should you attend the burial. I know what you two have been through since her diagnosis, and I know you have cared for her. I hate to think this is how it ends for you and her. You deserve better than that.

God bless you.

Njeri received an immediate response from Nil.

> *No thanks. I am standing by the decision I made at the courthouse yester-*
> *day. I tried discussing Lucy's funeral arrangement with you and Gloria*
> *well before Lucy's death. I am yielding to you and your family to get Lucy*
> *to her final resting plan. I am starting my healing process.*

As agreed during the court hearing, Njeri and Gloria went over to their law-yer's office to receive Lucy's personal belongings as ordered by the court. They arrived on time, only to be told that Nil had called saying he was late. Nil pulled up in a U-Haul, opened it, and the sisters saw the boxes. Nil handed Njeri a passport.

"We need her Kenyan passport, too," Gloria said.

"I don't have it, and I am not talking to you," Nil responded.

"We can't take her home without documents. Lucy kept her American passport and Kenyan passport together. We know because she told us. Njeri, he needs to give us Lucy's documents; otherwise, we will have problems."

When it seemed as though there was about to be a confrontation, Njeri spoke to Gloria in Kikuyu. "*Tigana nake, reke twarie na lawyer,*" which trans-lates, "Leave him alone. Let's talk to the lawyer."

There were too many boxes to fit into Njeri's and Gloria's vehicles. The sisters told the law firm's receptionist that they would rent a truck to pick up the boxes later. Nil, in a surprising act of kindness, offered to deliver the boxes to Njeri's house. Nil used a loading trolley to remove the boxes from the truck into Njeri's garage. He didn't say a word. When he was done, Njeri thanked him, but he ignored her and left. Gloria and Njeri looked at the boxes and felt a deep sadness. He must have packed these boxes a long time ago. There was no way he could have done it in two days. It was obvious that Nil had moved on, long before Lucy died.

The family had a week to come up with the funeral cost payment and the lawyer's fee, a total of $18,000. Tina, Lucy's faithful friend, led the fund-rais-ing effort at the Dumfries Health Center where Lucy had worked. Her other colleague, Samuel, posted a link to the YouCaring website on the Diaspora Messenger, which was picked up by Mwakilishi, newsletters that are widely popular with Kenyans around the world.

The Harambee concept was strange to some people. Some people did not understand why the family was insisting on taking Lucy's remains back to Kenya. One individual equated the process with begging and found it an inconvenience. "What is wrong with cremation?" some asked. Although the questions hurt, the sisters understood the cultural differences and explained that although the family was not against cremation, Lucy wished for her parents to bury her. In the end, the Harambee spirit was evident as the family raised more than $14,000 from Lucy's friends in California, family in England, Lucy's former colleagues, Njeri, Gloria, and Lydiah's friends from around the United States, the Kenyan Diaspora, and even strangers who were touched by Lucy's story on the YouCaring fund-raising website.

It was decided that the memorial service for Lucy's friends and family in the United States would be held on September 20, 2014. Pastor Lewis, who had spent a lot of time in the hospital with Lucy, was going to officiate. Njeri requested that Pastor Njoroge, a Kenyan pastor, who had visited and prayed with the family daily since Lucy's death, assist with the service as a family representative. Lucy's friends and family remembered her fondly during the long service. They were able to view the body for the last time. Lucy wore an off-white outfit with high heels to match, the last pair she had bought and never worn. Her hair and makeup were perfect. Njeri had requested that no one take pictures, and everyone obliged. After the service, friends and family gathered at Njeri's house for the repast. Pastor Lewis and his church had provided the food, enough for everyone. Tamara's daughter Kasaundra had stayed at the house and set up the meal beautifully buffet style. No one from Nil's family attended the service or the repast. The event was completely free of drama.

CHAPTER 25
Going Home

IN AN EFFORT TO FIND documents for Lucy, the sisters had to go through all the boxes, taking notes of the contents. It was obvious that Nil had decided to ignore some of the instructions in the court order. More importantly, the funeral home was having difficulty getting clearance to transport Lucy's body to Kenya because there was no proof that she was a Kenyan citizen. Gloria put together an e-mail to Ms. Boyd, their lawyer, asking that she send a request to Nil's lawyer for items that belonged to them and those that they knew Lucy wanted them to have. Ms. Boyd sent an e-mail to Nil's lawyer:

Nil delivered the bulk of the items on Friday, but my client reports there are a few things missing. They are the following:

1. *Two red chairs that my clients husband bought and Lucy painted*
2. *A glass bowl for her sister Lydiah*
3. *A big plant pot Lucy was holding for Njeri*
4. *Women's devotional Bible*
5. *Personal journals (diaries)*
6. *Expired Kenyan passport—this is required to transport her to Kenya*
7. *Kenyan birth certificate—this is proof she has dual citizenship*
8. *Expired American passport with Lucy's first husband's name*
9. *Naturalization certificate*
10. *Diamond and white gold earrings—given to Lucy by her ex-husband*
11. *Several watches*
12. *A gold necklace with a cross that Njeri gave to her*

If these items could be sent to my office as soon as possible, my client will pick them up.
Nil's lawyer responded immediately by writing:

PLEASE REMEMBER:

1.   *The reason we were in court was your clients' concern about Lucy's fu-neral and burial. There was no dispute among "next of kin" because her husband is her only next of kin. Nevertheless, he graciously gave place to their desires to honor her extended family; and*
2.   *He is her only heir at law and inherits all property from her. Once again, he graciously agreed to deliver some personal belongings which were spe-cifically defined in the consent order. To the extent that your clients are requesting things outside that list, they simply have no right to them.*

Notes of items 1–12 in your letter

1.   *The chairs belong to Nil.*
2.   *He doesn't know what glass bowl this is. Of course, it would belong to him. He probably wouldn't object but can't tell what this means.*
3.   *A plant pot. Also outside the order, but he wouldn't object.*
4.   *Already delivered*
5.   *He could not find any.*
6.   *He couldn't find it.*
7.   *He could not find it.*
8.   *He is not aware this exists. He gave the current passport.*
9.   *He could not find that.*
10. *He has delivered all the jewelry he could find.*
11. *He found a couple of watches, and they may have them.*
12. *Unless it was in the jewelry boxes that have been delivered, he doesn't have it.*

Because they recently moved in June, some things are in boxes. He has looked through everything, including unpacked boxes, in order to comply

*with the agreed order. While he will continue to look and to report any-
thing that he finds, I think your clients should assume he won't find more.*

After receiving Nil's lawyer's e-mail from Ms. Boyd, the sisters decided that
it was too costly and a waste of time to return to court and ask that Nil be
forced to give back Lucy's documents. The next business day morning, Njeri
and Tony went by the Metropolitan/Capital Funeral Service, which had been
contracted to send Lucy home; they were given the package, which included
a death certificate, a letter showing transportation requirements of an encased
container and that embalmment was done, a letter stating the Lucy did not
die of a communicable disease, and an out-of-state transit permit.

While sympathetic, the Kenyan embassy told Njeri and Tony that they
could not assist without any documents showing that Lucy was a Kenyan
citizen. Njeri sat at the visa room in tears, not knowing what to do. The
gentleman at the visa window called an embassy staff that came in to speak
to Njeri. Njeri explained her dilemma to the Kenyan Consular officer. The
officer was kind and consoling and told Njeri that there was a way to get
Lucy's body back to Kenya, but the Kenyan family would have to be actively
involved. The officer noted that the last time Lucy traveled in Kenya, she had
presented her expired Kenyan passport and the officers had noted the reference number in her American passport. The officer explained that this was a
good thing because the family in Kenya could go to Nyayo House in Nairobi
to track the record.

The sisters had kept details of Lucy's missing documents and the court
case from Mami and Baba. It was hard enough that they had lost a child and
were anxious to bring her home, but Mami was still suffering from the chemo
side effects, and the sisters felt it would be better to give her details face-to-
face. Njeri called her brother Jeff and explained that he needed to go to Nyayo
House to get Lucy's records. He also needed to get a letter from Baba, ac-
knowledging that indeed, Lucy was his child and he did not object having her
returned to Kenya for burial. Jeff would take all the documents to the ministry of foreign affairs to have them communicate with the Kenyan Embassy
in Washington, DC, giving OK to a clearance. To get all these expedited,

Njeri called her friend Fred, who was in Nairobi, and asked if he knew anyone in the Ministry of Foreign Affairs who could help. Fred coordinated the maneuverings of Jeff through Nyayo House and the ministry, and within a day, all the paperwork was completed. Sang, the other old friend from Kenya, brought the case to the Kenyan Embassy in Washington, DC, and solicited help from the staff. Njeri received a call telling her she could get the paperwork to send Lucy home.

On September 22, 2014, Lucy's body left Dulles Airport in Washington, DC, and arrived in Kenya on September 24, 2014. The burial ceremony was held on September 26, 2014, twenty days after her death.

CHAPTER 26

Lucy's Final Wish Comes True

As is customary, family and friends had been gathering in Nairobi and Karatina since they learned of Lucy's death. They were planning the funeral details and collecting money to cover the cost. In Nairobi, a relative offered meeting rooms in the city center as a venue at no charge. They raised enough money to cover the cost of all funeral expenses in Kenya. In Karatina, Mami and Baba had made a decision after the first weeks to suspend the daily meetings as they were unsure of when Lucy's body would arrive and wanted to grieve privately. The meetings in Karatina resumed when a date was set a week before the funeral. Funeral arrangements, program of events, and all other details were finalized before Lucy arrived in Kenya.

The KLM flight carrying Lucy's body arrived at Jomo Kenyatta International Airport in Nairobi just before 9:00 p.m.; her sisters Gloria, Lydiah, Nancy, and her brother Jeff were among multiple cousins and friends who had gone to the airport to receive her. After clearing with customs, the family followed the hearse to Montezuma Monalisa Funeral Home along Mbagathi Way in Nairobi. The staff at Montezuma was friendly and assured the family that they would provide all funeral services, including transporting Lucy to Karatina, located in the central province of Kenya, where Mami, Baba, and other relatives lived on the ancestral land.

Because of the distance and traffic in Nairobi, the family transported Lucy to Karatina the day before the funeral. Jeff and Wambugu, Lucy's nephew, rode in the hearse with Lucy and the driver. Gloria and Lydiah followed in a separate car. Mami and Baba had decided to wait until morning to go to the mortuary to see Lucy. The ride to Karatina took two and a half hours and arrived at Jamii Hospital Mortuary shortly before dark. After settling Lucy in, the family proceeded to Gitamaiyu, Baba's ancestral farm inherited through generations and where everyone as far as the eye could see was somehow related.

Njeri had stayed in Virginia to make sure the transportation went smoothly, that she was not in transit herself if anything went wrong. She arrived at Jomo Kenyatta International Airport after 10:00 p.m. and was met by her brother-in-law John, Gloria's former husband, who drove her to Karatina. When Njeri arrived at Mami and Baba's house after midnight, there was a group of women, including relatives and other villagers, preparing food. Njeri could not tell how many there were, but she was sure there were more than twenty. On the side of the house, young men were chatting, drinking beer, and listening to music. They had come to support Jeff.

Mami and Baba heard the car pull up the driveway and ran to the door to welcome their firstborn. Mami looked fragile. Her face had aged more than Njeri could remember. She was much thinner now and darker. Her eyes were sunken, hollow, and gray. She looked sad but managed to give Njeri a big smile and a hug. Njeri's aunt Tata Thiguku, Mami's younger sister, went to the kitchen to get her and John something to eat. Mami's older sister, Tata Ruguru, who was losing her eye sight and also had difficulty walking, rushed to embrace Njeri. Looking around, Njeri saw blankets and mattresses spread out everywhere; the house was completely full. It was 4:00 a.m. when they turned the lights off to go to bed because they all had to be at the funeral home by 9:00 a.m.

On that clear day, Njeri could see the peak of Mount Kenya from Gitamaiyu farm. Njeri woke up to find everyone else awake and having breakfast; it was 6:30 a.m. It gets quite cold in the morning in this part of Kenya, but those living there are used to the climate. The Ragati River, which originates from Mount Kenya, passes through Gitamaiyu farm, but as it was just before the short rainy season, the river was not as impressive as it normally was. Some young people decided to freshen up at the river. Inside the house, there was a line waiting for the shower. Outside, there was a big fire burning, with a big pot of hot water boiling on top. Several people were carrying buckets of cold water and would get a scoop of the hot water to wash their faces.

By 8:30 a.m., there were more than a hundred people congregated at Gitamaiyu farm. The funeral committee had rented passager vans to transport people to the funeral home. There were hundreds of people waiting at the funeral home to view Lucy's body.

Mami, Baba, and their children were led to the open casket to view the body. Baba stopped before he reached the blue casket and froze. "I can't do it," he told Mami. "I am not supposed to be burying my child."

Njeri noticed that Baba looked like he was going to pass out. This look was familiar, as she had seen it when Shiku died in 2008. Then, Njeri had asked another relative to take Baba out for fresh air. Baba could not look at Lucy in the casket. He held on to her picture that was placed on top of the casket and then sat down. Mami made her way to the front, supported by two of her nieces with Njeri, Gloria, Nancy, and Jeff in front. Mami reached out and touched Lucy's face. She kissed her on the forehead and then carefully straightened out Lucy's necklace.

"*Wui, mwana wakwa, kahiana maraika. Huroka mami.*" (Oh, my child, she looks like an angel. Rest mami). Mami stood silently for a long time. She looked intently at Lucy and, once in a while, would touch her. After what seemed like a long time, Mami turned around and said, "*Ni wandiga mwana wakwa. Ithui niithui tugagukora.*" (You have left me, my child. We are the ones to follow.) Mami walked over to where Baba was sitting and sat quietly next to him. The viewing procession continued with more people arriving. It took two hours before the master of ceremony decided to close the casket. Mami walked over one last time to see her child; this time, Baba followed quietly. They returned to their seats, wiping their eyes with handkerchiefs.

They arrived at Gitamaiyu farm at 11:00 a.m. The committee responsible for logistics had set up three tents, one for the family, another for clergy, and the biggest one for relatives and friends. All of Lucy's relatives, young and old, those who knew her and those who had never met her, were there. The government representative welcomed everyone to the ceremony. As was the custom, committees had been set up to ensure every detail was covered and their leaders were given an opportunity to speak at the funeral. Koki, Lucy's nephew, had designed and printed the funeral program in both English and Kikuyu and included the eulogy, songs, and pictures chosen by Mami, Baba, Lucy's siblings.

After the church service, Lucy's cousins carried her casket to the burial site where she was laid to rest. Mami and Baba looked solemn as the casket was lowered. The family was led away to the house as young men covered the casket. About an hour later, everyone returned to the burial site to place flowers. Njeri, Gloria, and Lydiah watched appreciatively on the sidelines as people flocked in to pay their last respects.

After they laid their flowers, they huddled together, and Gloria said, "Can you imagine denying all these friends and relatives a chance to say good-bye?"

"No, I cannot," Lydiah and Njeri said simultaneously.

After the ceremony, food was served at the tents. Mami, her sisters, and other elderly people ate at the house. The conversation was about Lucy. Mami was telling them about the last conversation she had with Lucy on the morning that she died. "She asked me to let her go. So, I know there is a place that people go. I will see her again," Mami was saying.

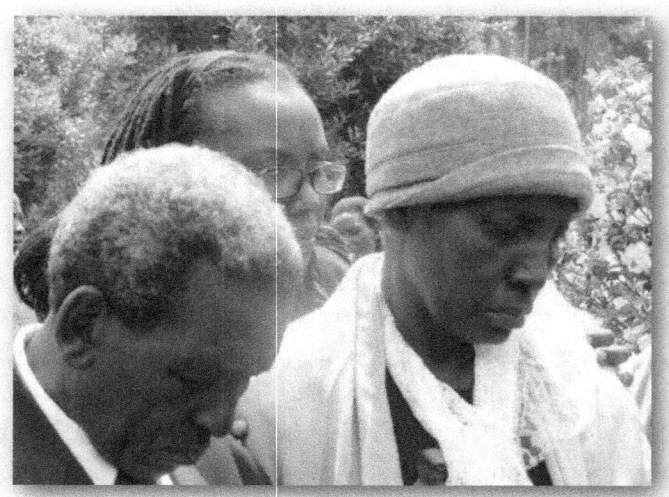

Mami and Baba looking down as Lucy's casket is lowered into the grave

CHAPTER 27

Finding Forgiveness

THE SISTERS RETURNED TO THE United States on separate dates. Lydiah, who had been in Kenya the longest, left first, followed by Gloria, then Njeri, who left on October 3, her late sister Shiku's birthday. Njeri's flight left at 8:00 a.m., which meant she had to leave Karatina in the wee hours of the morning. That night, Mami asked Njeri to sleep on the bed with her. Njeri thought it was a great idea; it would keep her from oversleeping, since the driver was scheduled to pick her up at 3:00 a.m. Before falling asleep, Mami spoke to Njeri as she always did.

"I was not able to complete school because of my pregnancy, but you and your siblings have done it for me. I am so proud of all of you. You are the oldest, and you have set a great example for your sisters and brother. It has been tough these past years, but you have all remained strong. Never forget that you are a family, and you must always support one another. Don't let anything come between you. You and Baba Ethel will be fine, no matter what comes your way.

"I know Nil mistreated Lucy. I want to call him on the phone and let him know what's on my mind, but he will probably laugh at my English, so, instead, I will write him a letter. He thinks he won because he got Lucy's things and insurance money, and now he thinks he has a woman of his dreams, but one day he will realize that material things are just that. One comes to this world with nothing and leaves with nothing. The way one treats others and saving your soul from bad actions is what is important in this world. Lucy lived a short but full life. She was happy when giving to family and strangers, so she lived a happy life. The happiest people in the world are those who do good things to others, so never stop giving and make sure your Ethel and Jazmine and all the children know that. The Bible tells us to forgive others so we can be forgiven. Please forgive Nil for making this difficult for you; you must move on. It's all in God's hands.

"You saw how many people came to celebrate Lucy. I am so proud of you and your sisters for bringing her back to me. Let all your friends in America know that we are grateful. You have all the people you need in your life, so don't waste time with those who want to hurt you or don't have your best interest; instead, pray for them. Show love to those you care about. We have to get up early, so let's go to sleep."

Mami woke Njeri up at 2:00 a.m. After a quick shower, Njeri sat down with Baba and Mami and enjoyed a cup of chai and *nduma*. The driver arrived at 4:00 a.m. Baba said a prayer before hugging Njeri good-bye. Mami held Njeri tight and kissed her several times, saying in English over and over again "I love you." Njeri took a quick selfie with Mami and Baba, rushed to Lucy's and Shiku's resting places to say good-bye, then got into the taxi and left. That was the last time Njeri saw Mami.

The first thing the sisters wanted to do after returning to the United States was thank family, friends, and everyone in the Kenyan Diaspora for their help in sending Lucy back to Kenya. The letter sent to the Diaspora Messenger newsletter said:

> *We the family of John and Esther Gathungu, would like to express our deep appreciation and sincere thanks for your kindness after the loss of our beloved Lucy. Your prayers, visits, donations, e-mails, and phone calls provided great comfort in our time of grief.*
>
> *We thank Dr. Verma and the entire team at Fort Belvoir Community Hospital who cared for Lucy over the years. We thank the management and staff of Dumfries Health Center who supported Lucy during her employment and after her passing. We would like to thank the clergy at Fort Belvoir, Reverend Father Opara, and Chaplain (MAJ) Nobles who*

ministered to Lucy and our family from the time she was admitted until her final moments. We would like to thank Pastor and Mrs. Lewis who were introduced to Lucy while she was admitted and took the lead in her funeral service in Virginia. We would like to thank A. L. Bennett and Son Funeral Home in Fredericksburg for their professionalism and support during a very complicated time. We would like to thank the immigration staff at the Kenya Embassy in Washington, DC.

We send our sincere gratitude to Kenyans in the Diaspora, most who did not know Lucy but donated funds that enabled us to honor her wish to be buried at home. Your donations through YouCaring continue to soften the financial worry. We especially thank Mr. Samuel, Mr. Sang, Mr. and Mrs. Arungah, Mr. Onyango, Mrs. Loyce, Pastor Njoroge, Mr. and Mrs. Adam Abdul Rahman, Kenyan Women Support Group led by Ms. Kiarie, and Mr. Kariuki of Diaspora Messenger. We particularly thank many of our friends and family who are not mentioned here by name; we know who you are and so does our good Lord.

We want to acknowledge and appreciate our family and friends in Kenya, especially all Thamaini and Githinji families, Dr. and Mrs. Githaiga, our church families, and all who contributed in cash and kind and without whom Lucy's journey home would not have been complete.

Our family will forever be grateful. We pray that "the Lord bless you and keep you; the Lord make his face shine on you and be gracious to you; the Lord turn his face toward you and give you peace" (Numbers 6:24–26).

On December 24, 2014, Mami suffered a brain aneurism after her morning shower and was rushed to the hospital in Karatina. She was still speaking coherently. She asked everyone to forgive her if she had wronged them. After several hours at Jamii Hospital in Karatina, the decision was made to transport her by ambulance to Nairobi to get adequate care. Mami was turned away at M. P. Shah hospital because a cash deposit of three thousand dollars could not be made prior to her admission. It was Christmas Eve and banks were closed. There was no way to send that kind of money, and the hospital would not take a credit card payment. Mami ran out of oxygen while Jeff and the ambulance driver drove around looking for a hospital that would admit Mami. Njeri's cousin, Wagwama, made several calls to different hospitals and promised to have the money in as soon as possible; Coptic Hospital on Ngong Road agreed to admit her in the intensive care unit. By the time Jeff and Mami reached the Coptic Hospital, Mami was in a coma. Mami passed away twelve days later on January 4, 2015. It was less than four months after Lucy's death; for the family, the grief was unbearable.

Once again, with the help of family and close friends, with sizeable cash donations from Rosslyn, Rae, Sang, Fred, Njeri, Loyce, Chris, Samuel, Wambui, Rachel, and many others in the Kenyan Diaspora, Gloria, Lydiah, and Njeri left the United States to attend Mami's funeral in Kenya. Mami was laid next to her two daughters, Shiku and Lucy. Nothing made sense.

A day after Mami's funeral, Jeff found a handwritten note in her handbag. She had told Jeff that she was writing a letter to Nil and wanted him to mail it. In it, Mami wrote that she knew Nil thought Lucy's family was poor, useless, and uneducated. She wrote that just like Lucy, she was a Christian who believed in a living God, and revenge was His. Mami concluded that she was OK and strong and that one day when her time came, she would follow Lucy and meet her in heaven. Everyone is a visitor passing by here on earth, Mami concluded in the letter. When Njeri returned to the United States, she mailed the letter to Nil's last known address.

For the family, Mami's last words and letter gave them permission to forgive Nil. They did not want to have any contact with him and were sure he felt the same. It didn't matter that he kept Lucy's journals, pictures, manuscript, and other things she wanted them to have; after all, they were just things. To her family, Lucy had a full, meaningful life. She taught her family and others great lessons that Nil could never take away from them. When the sisters looked back after Mami's death, they realized that if Nil had not acted the way he did, perhaps Lucy would not have completed her will asking to be buried in Kenya. This would have allowed Nil to do whatever he wanted with her remains against her wishes. His deplorable actions paved the way for the sisters to see Mami when they went to Kenya to bury Lucy. The sisters realized that Nil had not failed Lucy; he had failed as a man. The sisters felt nothing but pity for him. Indeed, Nil's infidelity and abuse, although disgusting, were a blessing in disguise. Those last days shared with Mami were some of the most cherished in the sisters' lives.

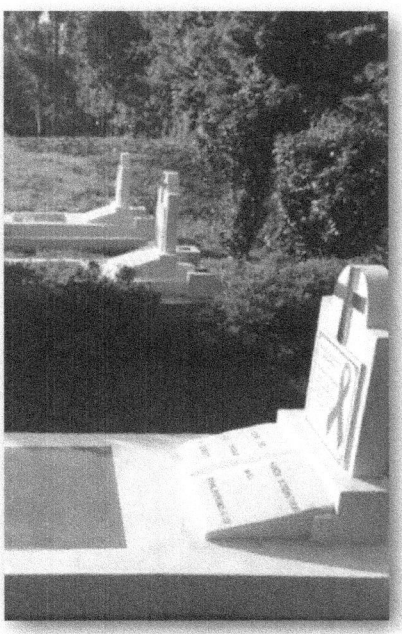

Lucy, Shiku and Mami

CONCLUSION

AT THE TIME OF THIS writing, nine years have passed since Shiku died and two years since Lucy's and Mami's deaths. Njeri, Gloria, Lydiah, and the rest of the family know that time does not heal everything—at least not yet—but time allows for sorrow to slowly fade. Smiles and laughter have replaced tears and sadness whenever they think of Shiku, Lucy, and Mami. The life lessons learned from these deaths are appreciated.

As Lucy said, "The truth is everyone will die. Each one living today will most likely be dead in the next one hundred years." Creating memories for loved ones has become a pastime for Lucy's family; they remember that during her last days, she longed for a chance to spend time experiencing life and places with them. They know life can change in an instant, so they view every day as precious. They share and celebrate minor accomplishments and minor setbacks. Among many lessons, Lucy taught them that bad things happen, but it's how one reacts that matters. They also learned that sometimes one has to make very difficult, unpopular choices, but as long as the choices are defensible, it's important to support the one making those choices and to understand they are not made lightly. At least once a month, the family is joined by their positive, uplifting, and supportive friends to socialize as Lucy wanted. They cook, eat, dance, talk, and make memories for one another, remembering Lucy's lesson that no matter what one is going through, someone else has it worse.

Lucy's vision of helping children in Kenya and educating people about colon cancer is clear not only to her family but to others who support the "Lucy's Blue Ribbon" project. The dream to support colon-cancer research and build a library in honor of Lucy for some very deserving underprivileged children in

Kenya is a big one. As Baba would tell his girls when they were young, "It is better to try and fail than not to try at all." The sisters will never stop trying to achieve Lucy's—and now their—dream.

A blue ribbon is the symbol for colon cancer. "Lucy's blue ribbon" was and still is representative of her faith, her struggle, her courage, her compassion, her generosity, her sense of humor, her hard work, her stubbornness, her determination, and her love for family and others. These qualities of Lucy will never die.

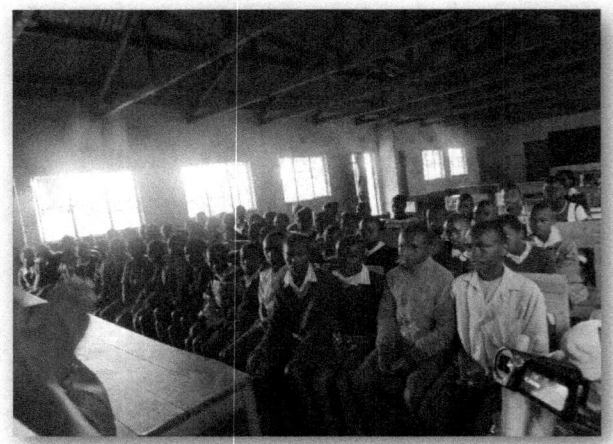

Lucy's Blue Ribbon future

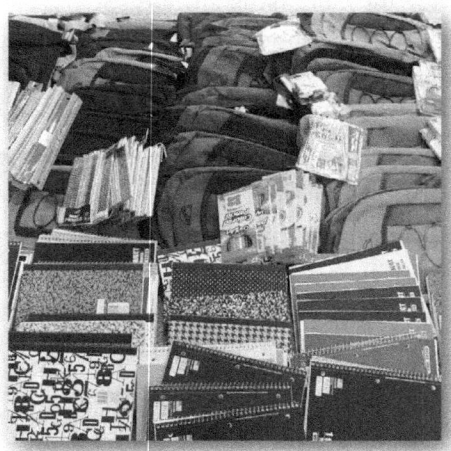

Some of the school supplies donated by friends for the children

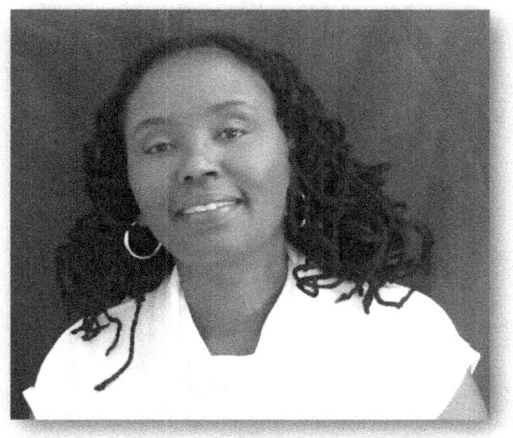

NJERI G. MOORE WAS BORN in Kenya and first moved to the United States in 1986 as a Pan American flight attendant. Moore eventually emigrated from her homeland permanently in 1990. She attended George Mason University in Fairfax, Virginia, and currently works as a federal employee in Washington, DC.

Moore founded the Lucy's Blue Ribbon Project to continue with her sister's vision for compassion and helping others. When she is not at her job, Moore enjoys spending time with her immediate and extended family, reading, cooking, and travelling. She currently lives in Virginia with her husband and is the mother of two girls.